Chiari I Malformation

Editors

JEFFREY RUSSELL LEONARD
DAVID D. LIMBRICK Jr

NEUROSURGERY
CLINICS OF NORTH AMERICA

www.neurosurgery.theclinics.com

Consulting Editors
RUSSELL LONSER
ISAAC YANG

October 2015 • Volume 26 • Number 4

ELSEVIER

1600 John F. Kennedy Boulevard • Suite 1800 • Philadelphia, Pennsylvania, 19103-2899

http://www.theclinics.com

NEUROSURGERY CLINICS OF NORTH AMERICA Volume 26, Number 4
October 2015 ISSN 1042-3680, ISBN-13: 978-0-323-40092-3

Editor: Jennifer Flynn-Briggs
Developmental Editor: Colleen Viola

Neurosurgery Clinics of North America (ISSN 1042-3680) is published quarterly by Elsevier Inc., 360 Park Avenue South, New York, NY 10010-1710. Months of issue are January, April, July, and October. Business and Editorial Offices: 1600 John F. Kennedy Blvd., Suite 1800, Philadelphia, PA 19103-2899. Customer Service Office: 11830 Westline Industrial Drive, St. Louis, MO 63146. Periodicals postage paid at New York, NY, and additional mailing offices. Subscription prices are $380.00 per year (US individuals), $572.00 per year (US institutions), $415.00 per year (Canadian individuals), $711.00 per year (Canadian institutions), $525.00 per year (international individuals), $711.00 per year (international institutions), $185.00 per year (US students), and $255.00 per year (international and Canadian students). International air speed delivery is included in all *Clinics* subscription prices. All prices are subject to change without notice. **POSTMASTER:** Send address changes to *Neurosurgery Clinics of North America*, Elsevier Periodicals Customer Service, 11830 Westline Industrial Drive, St. Louis, MO 63146. **Customer Service: 1-800-654-2452 (US and Canada). From outside the US and Canada, call: 1-314-453-7041. Fax: 1-314-453-5170. E-mail: JournalsCustomerService-usa@elsevier.com (for print support) and journalsonlinesupport-usa@elsevier.com (for online support).**

Reprints. For copies of 100 or more, of articles in this publication, please contact the Commercial Reprints Department, Elsevier Inc., 360 Park Avenue South, New York, NY 10010-1710. Tel. 212-633-3874; Fax: 212-633-3820; E-mail: reprints@elsevier.com.

Neurosurgery Clinics of North America is covered in *MEDLINE/PubMed (Index Medicus)*, *EMBASE/Excerpta Medica, and Current Contents/Clinical Medicine (CC/CM)*.

Contributors

CONSULTING EDITORS

RUSSELL LONSER, MD
Professor and Chair, Department of
Neurological Surgery, The Ohio State
University Wexner Medical Center, Columbus,
Ohio

ISAAC YANG, MD
Attending Neurosurgeon, Assistant Professor,
Department of Neurosurgery, Director of
Medical Student Education, David Geffen
School of Medicine at UCLA, Jonsson
Comprehensive Cancer Center, University of
California Los Angeles, Los Angeles, California

EDITORS

JEFFREY RUSSELL LEONARD, MD
Neurosurgeon-in-Chief, Professor of
Neurological Surgery, Nationwide Children's
Hospital; Professor of Neurological Surgery, The
Ohio State Medical School, Columbus, Ohio

DAVID D. LIMBRICK Jr, MD, PhD
Associate Professor of Neurological Surgery
and Pediatrics, St. Louis Children's Hospital,
Washington University School of Medicine,
St. Louis, Missouri

AUTHORS

**RICHARD C.E. ANDERSON, MD, FACS,
FAAP**
Assistant Professor of Neurological Surgery,
Department of Neurosurgery, Morgan Stanley
Children's Hospital of New York, The
Neurologic Institute, Columbia University,
New York, New York

ULRICH BATZDORF, MD
Professor, Neurosurgery, Brain Research
Institute, University of California, Los Angeles,
Los Angeles, California

DOUGLAS L. BROCKMEYER, MD
Professor of Neurosurgery; Adjunct Professor
of Pediatrics; Chief, Division of Pediatric
Neurosurgery, Primary Children's Hospital,
University of Utah, Salt Lake City, Utah

THOMAS J. BUELL, MD
Neurosurgery Resident Physician, Department
of Neurosurgery, University of Virginia,
Charlottesville, Virginia

AKBAR FAKHRI, MD
Mallinckrodt Institute of Radiology,
Washington University School of Medicine,
St. Louis, Missouri

HANNAH E. GOLDSTEIN, MD
Department of Neurosurgery, Morgan
Stanley Children's Hospital of New York,
The Neurologic Institute, Columbia University,
New York, New York

MANU S. GOYAL, MD, MSc
Mallinckrodt Institute of Radiology,
Washington University School of Medicine,
St. Louis, Missouri

JACOB K. GREENBERG, MD, MSCI
Resident, Department of Neurological Surgery,
Washington University, St. Louis, Missouri

TENNER J. GUILLAUME, MD
Department of Orthopedic Surgery, Gillette
Children's Hospital, St. Paul, Minnesota

TODD C. HANKINSON, MD
Children's Hospital Colorado; Assistant
Professor, Department of Neurosurgery,
University of Colorado Anschutz Medical
Campus, Aurora, Colorado

JOHN D. HEISS, MD
Surgical Neurology Branch, National Institute
of Neurological Disorders and Stroke, National
Institutes of Health, Bethesda, Maryland

JOHN A. JANE Jr, MD
Director, Division of Pediatrics; Professor of
Neurosurgery and Pediatrics, Department of
Neurological Surgery, University of Virginia
Health Science Center, Charlottesville, Virginia

JAMES M. JOHNSTON Jr, MD
Assistant Professor, Division of Pediatric
Neurosurgery, Department of Neurosurgery,
Children's of Alabama, University of Alabama
at Birmingham, Birmingham, Alabama

ELYNE N. KAHN, MD
Department of Neurosurgery, University of
Michigan, Ann Arbor, Michigan

MICHAEL P. KELLY, MD, MSc
Assistant Professor of Orthopedic and
Neurological Surgery, Department of
Orthopedic Surgery, Washington University
School of Medicine, St. Louis, Missouri

ALEXANDER KSENDZOVSKY, MD
Department of Neurological Surgery, University
of Virginia Health Science Center,
Charlottesville, Virginia

LAWRENCE G. LENKE, MD
Professor of Orthopedic and Neurological
Surgery, Department of Orthopedic Surgery,
Washington University School of Medicine,
St. Louis, Missouri

CORMAC O. MAHER, MD
Department of Neurosurgery, University of
Michigan, Ann Arbor, Michigan

KARIN M. MURASZKO, MD
Department of Neurosurgery, University of
Michigan, Ann Arbor, Michigan

WALTER JERRY OAKES, MD
Professor, Department of Neurosurgery,
University of Alabama at Birmingham,
Birmingham, Alabama

EDWARD H. OLDFIELD, MD
Professor of Neurological Surgery and Internal
Medicine, Director of Neuro-endocrine,
Department of Neurosurgery, University of
Virginia, Charlottesville, Virginia

TAE SUNG PARK, MD
Shi H. Huang Professor of Neurological
Surgery, Professor of Pediatrics and Anatomy
and Neurobiology, Neurosurgeon-in-Chief,
St. Louis Children's Hospital; Department of
Neurological Surgery, Washington University,
St. Louis, Missouri

JONATHAN PINDRIK, MD
Fellow, Division of Pediatric Neurosurgery,
Children's of Alabama, University of
Alabama at Birmingham, Birmingham,
Alabama

ISAAC JONATHAN POMERANIEC, BSc
Department of Neurological Surgery, University
of Virginia Health Science Center,
Charlottesville, Virginia

THOMAS RIDDER, MD
Children's Hospital Colorado, Aurora,
Colorado

BRANDON G. ROCQUE, MD, MS
Assistant Professor, Department of
Neurosurgery, University of Alabama at
Birmingham, Birmingham, Alabama

MANISH N. SHAH, MD
Departments of Pediatric Surgery and
Neurosurgery, University of Texas, Health
Science Center at Houston, Houston, Texas

HEATHER S. SPADER, MD
Division of Pediatric Neurosurgery, Primary
Children's Hospital, University of Utah, Salt
Lake City, Utah

R. SHANE TUBBS, PhD
Seattle Science Foundation, Seattle,
Washington

CHESTER K. YARBROUGH, MD, MPHS
Chief Resident, Department of Neurological
Surgery, Washington University, St. Louis,
Missouri

PEARL L. YU, MD
Department of Neurological Surgery, University
of Virginia Health Science Center,
Charlottesville, Virginia

Contents

Current understanding of the hindbrain hernias known as Chiari I malformations is based on more than 100 years of pathologic and clinical experience. Over time, the definition of this finding has been analyzed and altered. The term Chiari I malformation is currently used to describe tonsillar ectopia in a wide range of patients with varying embryonic derailments. This article discusses this malformation, its various definitions, and varied anatomic traits. In addition, the morphology of the commonly associated syringomyelia is reviewed.

This article summarizes the current understanding of the pathophysiology of the Chiari I malformation that is based on observations of the anatomy visualized by modern imaging with MRI and prospective studies of the physiology of patients before and after surgery. The pathogenesis of a Chiari I malformation of the cerebellar tonsils is grouped into 4 general mechanisms.

Chiari I malformation (CM) is a common neurosurgical diagnosis, and spinal cord syrinx is frequently found in patients with CM. Asymptomatic CM is a common imaging finding. Symptomatic CM is less common. Variation in prevalence estimates may be attributed to differences in sensitivity of CM detection between studies as well as differences in the populations being analyzed. The prevalence of low tonsil position and CM on MRI is higher in children and young adults compared with older adults. Studies that include a large number of older adults find a lower prevalence compared with analyses of children.

Chiari I malformation and syringomyelia may be associated with a wide spectrum of symptoms and signs in children. Clinical presentations vary based on patient age and relative frequency; some diagnoses represent incidental radiographic findings. Occipitocervical pain, propagated or intensified by Valsalva maneuvers (or generalized irritability in younger patients unable to communicate verbally), and syringomyelia with or without scoliosis are the most common clinical presentations. Cranial nerve or brainstem dysfunction also may be observed in younger patients and is associated with more complex deformity that includes ventral compression secondary to basilar invagination, retroflexion of the dens, and/or craniocervical instability.

the hindbrain is often recommended. In young patients (<10 years old) and/or those with small coronal Cobb measurements (<40°), decompression of the hindbrain may lead to resolution of the spinal deformity. Spinal fusion is reserved for those curves that progress to deformities greater than 50°. Further research is needed to understand the underlying pathophysiology to improve prognostication and treatment of this patient population.

NEUROSURGERY CLINICS OF NORTH AMERICA

Erratum

In the July 2015 issue (Volume 26, number 3) of *Neurosurgery Clinics*, for the articles "Endoscopic Endonasal Approach For Removal Of Tuberculum Sellae Meningiomas" and "The Endoscopic Endonasal Approach For Removal Of Petroclival Chondrosarcomas," Amin Kassam, MD was inadvertently omitted from the author list.

http://dx.doi.org/10.1016/j.nec.2015.08.001
1042-3680/15/$ – see front matter

Preface
Chiari I Malformation: Adult and Pediatric Considerations

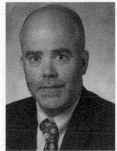
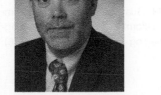

Jeffrey Russell Leonard, MD   David D. Limbrick Jr, MD, PhD

Editors

Chiari type I malformation (CM-1) is encountered across the full spectrum of neurosurgical practice, affecting patients from infancy through adulthood. As with any neurosurgical disorder, understanding the pathophysiology, clinical presentation, and radiographic findings is paramount in determining the appropriate management approach for any given patient with CM-1. The objective of this issue of *Neurosurgery Clinics of North America*, titled "Chiari I Malformation," is to provide this critical information in a single, concise volume with up-to-date reports from leading experts in the field of CM-1.

While there is general acknowledgment that CM-1 is characterized by cerebellar tonsillar ectopia, there remains no consensus definition of the disorder. Indeed, large institutional studies have shown that ~3% of children and 1% of adults demonstrate radiographic evidence of CM-1, yet the conditions under which such radiographic findings translate to clinically significant CM-1 are unclear.[1,2] Furthermore, tonsillar ectopia also may be associated with any number of developmental and acquired disorders (eg, craniofacial syndromes, hydrocephalus, posterior fossa tumors). Thus, a clear understanding of the clinical presentation of CM-1 in both pediatric and adult patients has direct bearing on both patient selection and the approach for operative management.

This issue contains detailed descriptions of the surgical treatment of CM-1, with photos and videos showing posterior fossa decompression in stepwise fashion with expert technical details and operative nuances. These will undoubtedly be of interest to all neurosurgical audiences, from trainees to senior surgeons. There is also thorough consideration of operative risks and complications as well as treatment efficacy and need for additional, advanced neurosurgical procedures, for example, in cases of the "complex Chiari," such as occipital-cervical fusion or ventral decompression.

Advances in the field of CM-1 have been closely linked to the implementation of novel imaging techniques, and it is expected that the development and application of new MRI protocols enabling detailed investigation of cerebrospinal fluid hydrodynamics, craniovertebral junction anatomy, and spinal cord and brainstem white matter tracts will facilitate our growing understanding of the pathophysiology and treatment of CM-1. Of particular importance in advancing CM-1 is the development of improved clinical outcomes instruments, those that are specific for CM-1 and place emphasis on patient-centered outcomes and quality of life. Using such instruments to track outcomes in large numbers of patients enrolled across multi-institutional clinical

Neurosurg Clin N Am 26 (2015) xiii–xiv
http://dx.doi.org/10.1016/j.nec.2015.07.002
1042-3680/15/$ – see front matter © 2015 Published by Elsevier Inc.

research networks will greatly facilitate our ability to optimize the care of patients with CM-1.

Jeffrey Russell Leonard, MD
Nationwide Children's Hospital
The Ohio State Medical School
700 Children's Drive
Columbus, OH 43205, USA

David D. Limbrick Jr, MD, PhD
Department of Neurosurgery
St. Louis Children's Hospital
Washington University School of Medicine
One Children's Place, Suite 4S20
St Louis, MI 63110, USA

E-mail addresses:
Jeffrey.Leonard@nationwidechildrens.org (J.R. Leonard)
limbrickd@wustl.edu (D.D. Limbrick)

REFERENCES

1. Strahle J, Muraszko KM, Kapurch J, et al. Chiari malformation Type 1 and syrinx in children undergoing magnetic resonance imaging. J Neurosurg Pediatr 2011;8(2):205–13.
2. Meadows J, Kraut M, Guarnieri M, et al. Asymptomatic Chiari Type I malformations identified on magnetic resonance imaging. J Neurosurg 2000;92(6): 920–6.

Definitions and Anatomic Considerations in Chiari I Malformation and Associated Syringomyelia

CrossMark

R. Shane Tubbs, PhD

KEYWORDS

- Anatomy • Hindbrain hernia • Tonsillar ectopia • Neurosurgery • Syrinx • Chiari malformation

KEY POINTS

- Understanding of the Chiari I malformation has evolved over time.
- The Chiari I malformation has many different known and unknown causes.
- The definition of the Chiari I malformation is in need of refinement based on continued clinical and surgical experience.

INTRODUCTION

Since the original description and classification of hindbrain hernias more than a century ago,[1,2] the Chiari malformations have revealed much of their pathophysiology and have become easily diagnosed radiologically. With the availability of MRI, more and more patients are being diagnosed but without symptoms or appropriate symptoms. Time and clinical experience have shed light on the edges of this diagnosis, but indications for surgical intervention in some patient groups have become indistinct.

The 4 traditional types of Chiari malformations represent various clinical and anatomic processes that entail involvement of the rhombencephalon (hindbrain). Chiari types I, II, and III involve varying degrees of herniation of rhombencephalic derivatives out of the posterior fossa. Chiari type IV malformations involve cerebellar hypoplasia or aplasia, with no herniation of the hindbrain. At present, there is no consensus on how to define, treat, or label a causal process for the pathologic term Chiari malformation. Although the Chiari classification is usually helpful in categorizing patients, this scheme probably does not represent a precise continuum of the same disease and does not provide the classification needed to compartmentalize all forms of hindbrain hernias encountered. Moreover, with regard to this article, multiple causes are responsible for the Chiari I malformation (CIM) (Fig. 1), which is an imprecise term, usually diagnosed on a single midline sagittal MRI image, that does not take into account respiration, presence or absence of Valsalva maneuver, shape or thickness of the foramen magnum, or that the cerebellar tonsils are paired parasagittal structures (Figs. 2 and 3).[3]

DEFINITION

In Chiari's original definition, the type I malformation was considered herniation of the cerebellar tonsils below the plane of the foramen magnum but the degree of herniation was not defined. Therefore, the precise definition of the type I malformation has been debated. In addition, Chiari malformations represent a wide range of anatomy

Disclosure: The author has no commercial or financial conflicts of interest and no funding was used for the production of this article.
Seattle Science Foundation, 550 17th Ave #600, Seattle, WA 98122, USA
E-mail address: shane.tubbs@childrensal.org

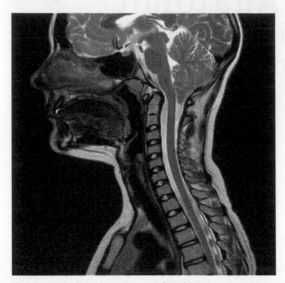

Fig. 1. Typical CIM on T2-weighted MRI.

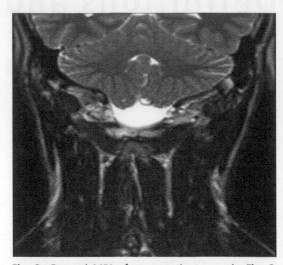

Fig. 3. Coronal MRI of same patient seen in **Fig. 2**, noting mild right-sided tonsillar ectopia that was not evident on sagittal imaging.

that may or may not have common embryologic origins. For example, the CIMs seen in patients with bony overgrowth of the posterior fossa, growth hormone deficiency, or craniosynostosis represent the same effect from varied causes. Therefore, the term CIM should be considered a generic appellation for a physical finding and should not imply a specific congenital cause.

In an attempt to better categorize tonsillar ectopia, Aboulezz and colleagues[4] retrospectively examined 95 cases. In normal controls, the cerebellar tonsils did not extend more than 3 mm below

the plane of the foramen magnum. These investigators considered herniation below 5 mm to be pathologic. Barkovich and colleagues[5] measured the position of the cerebellar tonsils with respect to the inferior aspect of the foramen magnum in 200 normal patients and in 25 patients with a diagnosis of CIM. In the normal group, the mean position of the tonsils was 1 mm above the foramen magnum with a range from 8 mm above the foramen magnum to 5 mm below. In the patients with CIM, the mean position was 13 mm below the foramen magnum with a range from 3 mm below the foramen magnum to 29 mm below. Fourteen percent of normal patients had tonsils extending slightly below the foramen magnum. With 2 mm below the foramen magnum taken as the lowest extent for tonsils in normal patients, the sensitivity in predicting symptomatic patients was 100% and the specificity was 98.5% (3 false-positives). When 3 mm below the foramen magnum was used as the lowest normal tonsillar position, the sensitivity was 96% and the specificity was 99.5%. In addition, Mikulis and colleagues[3] found that normal tonsils may prolapse up to 6 mm during the first 10 years of life and ascend gradually with increasing age.

ANATOMIC FINDINGS OF THE CHIARI I MALFORMATION

The CIM was originally described as caudal displacement of the cerebellar tonsils to a level below the plane of the foramen magnum. In general, 3 to 5 mm of caudal descent of the tonsils is considered a CIM.[5] There are other associated findings seen surgically, radiologically, and at

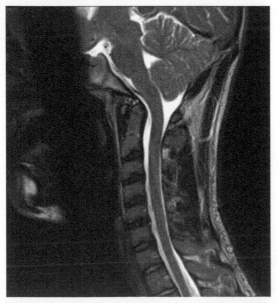

Fig. 2. Sagittal MRI without evidence of tonsillar ectopia.

postmortem in patients with CIM. These findings are described and categorized here according to their anatomic locations.

Skull

Basilar skull and craniocervical junction anomalies (eg, third occipital condyle) are seen in many patients with CIMs.[6–10] It is now appreciated that the supraocciput and exocciput are underdeveloped in many patients with CIMs, and there is shortening of the supraocciput. The clivus is also often shorter,[11] with a larger than normal foramen magnum, although in some diseases involving CIM, the foramen magnum may be smaller than normal.[7] The midline sagittal diameter of the foramen magnum, measured from basion to opisthion, ranged from 30 to 40 mm (mean, 36.7 mm) in an earlier study from our group.[12] On axial imaging, the maximal width of the foramen magnum was measured from 12 to 31 mm (mean, 26 mm). The foramen magnum may be narrowed in the coronal plane (ie, lateral compression).[13]

The posterior fossa is shallower in many patients with this type of malformation. It is now known that, like Chiari type II malformations, type I malformations often have smaller than normal posterior cranial fossa volumes.[11,12] Also, various forms of craniosynostosis are associated with CIM ostensibly because of reduced intracranial volume.[14]

Other basilar skull abnormalities seen with the CIM include empty sellae, clival concavities, basilar impression, large midline occipital keels, and remnants of the proatlas, such as an accessory occipital condyle.[6] The midline sagittal length of the baslocciput in this group has been measured with a range from 20 to 29 mm (mean, 24 mm).[8]

Spine

Klippel-Feil deformity and atlanto-occipital assimilation are two of the most common spinal defects in type I malformations.[6,8] Other occasional findings are retroflexion of the odontoid process (**Fig. 4**) and thickening of the ligamentum flavum. The posterior atlanto-occipital membrane may also be thickened. Another common entity seen in CIMs is scoliosis, which is usually caused by an underlying syrinx and is most likely to be a single curve with a convexity to the left. Scoliosis may be present in the absence of CIM.[15]

Retroflexion of the odontoid process is commonly seen in patients with CIM and most commonly in female patients.[16] Greater degrees of retroflexion have been correlated with a greater prevalence of syringomyelia.[16] This resultant anterior compression may contribute to symptoms

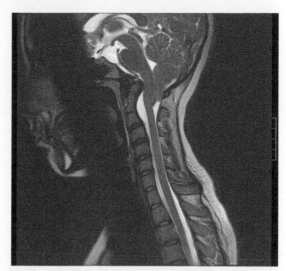

Fig. 4. Retroflexion of the odontoid in a patient with descent of the cerebellar tonsils and medulla oblongata; the so-called Chiari 1.5 malformation.

because of a compounded stenosis at the foramen magnum.[17]

Ventricles and Cisterns

Ventricular anatomy, other than an occasionally elongated fourth ventricle, is normal in CIM. Hydrocephalus has been described in 3% to 10% of this subgroup but the hindbrain hernia is secondary and should not be considered with this malformation as a whole (**Fig. 5**).[18,19] Note that,

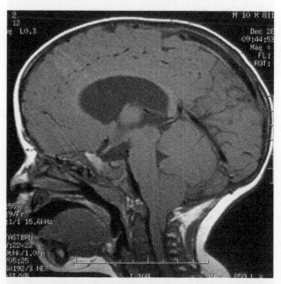

Fig. 5. Patient with hydrocephalus and tonsillar ectopia. Although this is often termed a CIM, it is a secondary effect and can resolve with intervention. Therefore, terming this a malformation is inappropriate.

in many of these patients, the retrocerebellar cerebrospinal fluid (CSF) spaces are obliterated or diminished.[19]

Fourth Ventricular Outlet Obstruction

Our group detailed the incidence of arachnoid veils found in juxtaposition with the foramen of Magendie in patients with hindbrain herniation (**Fig. 6**).[20] In addition, radiological studies were retrospectively reviewed in cases in which such an anomaly was noted intraoperatively. Of 140 patients with CIM who underwent decompressive surgery, an associated syrinx was shown in 80 (57%). The foramen of Magendie was obstructed by an arachnoid veil in 12.5% of these patients. On retrospective review of imaging studies, none of these anomalous structures was evident. In all patients with an arachnoid veil and syringomyelia resolution of syringomyelia was revealed on postoperative imaging.

Similar to arachnoid veils, the left and right posterior inferior cerebellar arteries may be touching (so-called kissing posterior inferior cerebellar arteries) at the foramen of Magendie and thus block CSF egress from the fourth ventricle with resultant syrinx formation.

Meninges

The slope of the tentorium cerebelli may be elevated in type I malformations.[19] In addition, thickening of the arachnoid at the level of the foramen magnum is routinely seen, and may be accompanied by a constricting dural band. Another thickened and constricting band of dura is occasionally found at the level of the posterior arch of the atlas.

Spinal Cord and Syringomyelia

The prominent spinal cord finding in type I malformations is a syrinx. Using MRI, cavitation of the cord has been reported in up to 75% of patients.[18,19,21–24] These syrinxes are usually found in the lower cervical and upper thoracic spinal cord. Syrinxes also often have a septated appearance (ie, haustra) (**Fig. 7**), which occurs less commonly in syrinxes caused by tumor, infection, tethered cord, or trauma. There is routinely a segment of cord that is spared (ie, skip area) from cavitation between the fourth ventricle and the beginning of the syrinx in the cervical cord.[18] This condition is seen most often in the cervical cord and frequently does not communicate with the fourth ventricle via a radiographically identifiable central canal or other syringeal pathway. There is currently no consensus on the correlation between the extent of tonsillar herniation and the presence of a syrinx. Syringomyelia can occur

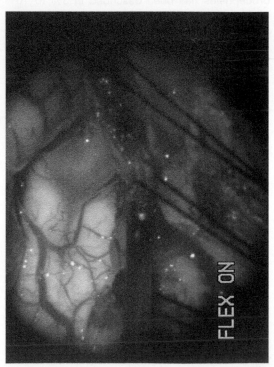

Fig. 6. Arachnoid veil seen covering the midline fourth ventricular outlet in a patient undergoing CIM decompression.

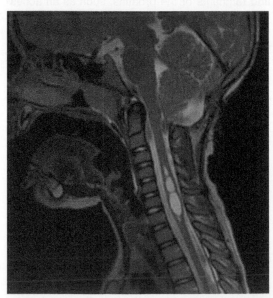

Fig. 7. Postoperative image in a patient with CIM and syringomyelia. Note the haustra (septations) within the syrinx, which usually indicates a hindbrain herniation cause for the fluid accumulation.

throughout the spinal cord, but syrinxes that spare the cervical spinal cord should be evaluated for a non-Chiari origin. The more distal in the spinal cord, the less likely it is that a syrinx is related to the CIM.

In an earlier study, our group[24] retrospectively reviewed radiological and operative data in 8 patients who continued to have syringomyelia following a decompressive procedure. Seven (88%) of these patients had complete resolution of their syrinxes following a second operation. At repeated operation, obstruction at the foramen of Magendie was seen in 6 patients. In 1 patient in whom the dura was not opened during the first operation, the second operation revealed an arachnoid veil that occluded the foramen of Magendie. No single radiological measurement was found to aid in the prediction of which patients would not respond to the first decompressive procedure. Furthermore, no operative finding was unique to any single patient. All but 1 patient in whom confirmation of a patent foramen of Magendie was made at repeated operation (ie, lysing of arachnoid veils, stent placement, unllateral tonsillar coagulation) had resolution of their syringomyelia.

Brain

Brainstem and cerebellar tonsils

With CIMs, the brain is generally free from anomalies other than the tonsillar herniation. In rare instances, the midbrain, pons, and medulla have been noted to be elongated, with occasional medullary kinking or flattening. The medulla oblongata may be displaced downward (discussed later). The herniated tonsils often lose their folial pattern and become atrophic from chronic compression. The cerebellar tonsillar tips are also often frankly ischemic and may degenerate into a cystic component.[25]

The cerebellar tonsils are usually described as peglike or pointed and are often asymmetric. Tips that are elongated and pointed are more likely to become symptomatic than are tips that are rounded and blunt. We measured the degree of left and right tonsillar herniation in 42 pediatric patients with a symptomatic CIM and made clinical/radiological correlations.[26] Eighteen percent of all patients with tonsillar asymmetry had clinical symptoms or physical findings referable to the inequality of their hindbrain herniation. In addition, 95% of patients with a coexisting syringomyelia had a right cerebellar tonsillar herniation greater than the left.

FORME FRUSTE
Chiari 1.5

Chiari 1.5 specifically describes patients with Chiari type I malformations but with the addition

of an elongated brainstem and fourth ventricle (see **Fig. 4**). Our group's earlier analysis of 22 patients found that the obex (measured on midsagittal MRI on a line from and perpendicular to the McRae line) was a mean of 14.4 mm inferior to the foramen magnum, and the medulla had a flattened appearance in the midsagittal plane in all patients.[27] Syringomyelia was documented in 50% of the cases. No abnormalities or caudal descent of the midbrain or pons was identified. Eighteen patients experienced resolution of preoperative symptoms. Persistence of syringomyelia prompted a second posterior fossa operation secondary to progressive scoliosis in 13.6% of the patients. No single sign or symptom was found to be peculiar to the Chiari 1.5 malformation, although all patients in whom this diagnosis was established had undergone a posterior fossa decompressive surgery.

Chiari 0

A small group of patients with CSF equilibrium changes at the craniocervical junction has been

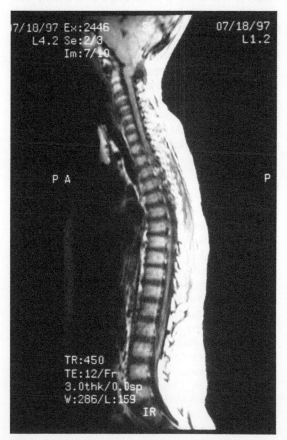

Fig. 8. Patient with concomitant CIM and lipomyelomeningocele.

said to have the type 0 malformation.[28] These patients have syringohydromyelia but minimal or no findings of hindbrain herniation when imaged, but may have intermittent caudal descent of the cerebellar tonsils with Valsalva maneuvers that is not captured on static imaging. This speculation is supported by the pulsatility caused by the cardiac cycle seen operatively and on dynamic imaging studies. In these patients and in order to verify this diagnosis, posterior fossa decompression must decrease the size of the syrinx. However, before recommending such a procedure, it is important to exclude other causes of syringomyelia. Many of the Chiari type 0 group have craniocervical anomalies such as those seen in the CIM and, genetically, have been found to be on the same continuum.[29] Operative findings include arachnoid veils and adhesions obstructing the foramen of Magendie and crowding the tissue at the foramen magnum.

SUMMARY

The hindbrain hernias known as the Chiari malformations represent a wide range of anatomy that may or may not have common embryologic origins. Even within the CIM classification, various embryonic derailments are probably at play. The tonsillar ectopia sometimes seen with various forms of craniosynostosis is not caused by the same processes that are involved with the tonsillar ectopia that is occasionally seen in patients with lipomyelomeningocele (**Fig. 8**).[30] Therefore, the definition of the CIM is in need of refinement based on continued clinical and surgical experience.[31]

REFERENCES

1. Chiari H. Uber Veranderungen des Kleinhirns infolge von Hydrocephalie des Grosshirns. Dtsch Med Wochenschr 1891;17:1172–5.
2. Chiari H. Uber Veranderungen des Kleinhirns, der Pons und der Medulla oblongata infolge von congenitaler Hydrocephalie des Grosshirns. Denkschr Akad Wiss 1895;63:71–115.
3. Mikulis DJ, Diaz O, Egglin TK, et al. Variance of the position of the cerebellar tonsils with age: preliminary report. Radiology 1992;183:725–8.
4. Aboulezz AO, Sartor K, Geyer CA, et al. Position of cerebellar tonsils in the normal population and in patients with Chiari malformation: a quantitative approach with MR imaging. J Comput Assist Tomogr 1985;9:1033–6.
5. Barkovich AJ, Wippold FJ, Sherman JL, et al. Significance of cerebellar tonsillar position of MR. AJNR Am J Neuroradiol 1986;7:795–9.
6. Menezes A. Primary craniovertebral anomalies and the hindbrain herniation syndrome (Chiari I): data base analysis. Pediatr Neurosurg 1995;23:260–9.
7. Schady W, Metcalfe RA, Butler P. The incidence of craniocervical body anomalies in the adult Chiari malformation. J Neurol Sci 1987;82:193–203.
8. Cesmebasi A, Loukas M, Hogan E, et al. The Chiari malformations: a review with emphasis on anatomical traits. Clin Anat 2015;28:184–94.
9. Cesmebasi A, Muhleman MA, Hulsberg P, et al. Occipital neuralgia: anatomic considerations. Clin Anat 2015;28:101–8.
10. Tubbs RS, Lingo PR, Mortazavi MM, et al. Hypoplastic occipital condyle and third occipital condyle: review of their dysembryology. Clin Anat 2013;26:928–32.
11. Stovner LJ, Bergan U, Nilsen G, et al. Posterior cranial fossa dimensions in the Chiari I malformation: relation to pathogenesis and clinical presentation. Neuroradiology 1993;35:113–8.
12. Tubbs RS, Hill M, Loukas M, et al. Volumetric analysis of the posterior cranial fossa in a family with four generations of the Chiari malformation Type I. J Neurosurg Pediatr 2008;1:21–4.
13. Tubbs RS, Chern JJ, Muhleman M, et al. Lateral compression of the foramen magnum with the Chiari I malformation: case illustrations. Childs Nerv Syst 2013;29:495–8.
14. Cinalli G, Renier D, Sebag G, et al. Chronic tonsillar herniation in Crouzon's and Apert's syndromes: the role of premature synostosis of the lambdoid suture. J Neurosurg 1995;83:575–82.
15. Tubbs RS, Doyle S, Conklin M, et al. Scoliosis in a child with CIM and the absence of syringomyelia: case report and a review of the literature. Childs Nerv Syst 2006;22:1351–4.
16. Tubbs RS, Wellons JC 3rd, Blount JP, et al. Inclination of the odontoid process in the pediatric Chiari I malformation. J Neurosurg 2003;98:43–9.
17. Grabb P, Mapstone T, Oakes W. Ventral brainstem compression in pediatric and young adult patients with Chiari I malformations. Neurosurgery 1999;44:520–8.
18. Tubbs RS, Beckman J, Naftel RP, et al. Institutional experience with 500 cases of surgically treated pediatric Chiari malformation Type I. J Neurosurg Pediatr 2011;7:248–56.
19. Milhorat T, Chou M, Trinidad E, et al. CIMs redefined: clinical and radiographic findings for 364 symptomatic patients. Neurosurgery 1999;44:1005–17.
20. Tubbs RS, Smyth MD, Wellons JC 3rd, et al. Arachnoid veils and the CIM. J Neurosurg 2004;100: 465–7.
21. Hendrix P, Griessenauer CJ, Cohen-Adad J, et al. Spinal diffusion tensor imaging: a comprehensive review with emphasis on spinal cord anatomy and clinical applications. Clin Anat 2015;28:88–95.

22. Arnautovic A, Splavski B, Boop FA, et al. Pediatric and adult Chiari malformation Type I surgical series 1965-2013: a review of demographics, operative treatment, and outcomes. J Neurosurg Pediatr 2015;15:161–77.

23. Oakes W. Chiari malformations and syringomyelia. In: Rengachary S, Wilkins R, editors. Principles of neurosurgery. London: Wolf Publishing; 1994. p. 9.1–9.18.

24. Tubbs RS, Webb DB, Oakes WJ. Persistent syringomyelia following pediatric Chiari I decompression: radiological and surgical findings. J Neurosurg 2004;100:460–4.

25. Stevenson CB, Leach JL, Gupta A, et al. Cystic degeneration of the cerebellar tonsils in pediatric patients with Chiari Type I malformation. J Neurosurg Pediatr 2009;4:557–63.

26. Tubbs RS, Wellons JC 3rd, Oakes WJ. Asymmetry of tonsillar ectopia in CIM. Pediatr Neurosurg 2002;37:199–202.

27. Tubbs RS, Iskandar BJ, Bartolucci AA, et al. A critical analysis of the Chiari 1.5 malformation. J Neurosurg 2004;101:179–83.

28. Iskandar BI, Hedlund GL, Grabb PA, et al. The resolution of syringomyelia without hindbrain herniation after posterior fossa decompression. J Neurosurg 1998;89:212–6.

29. Markunas CA, Tubbs RS, Moftakhar R, et al. Clinical, radiological, and genetic similarities between patients with Chiari Type I and Type 0 malformations. J Neurosurg Pediatr 2012;9:372–8.

30. Tubbs RS, Bui CJ, Rice WC, et al. Critical analysis of the Chiari malformation Type I found in children with lipomyelomeningocele. J Neurosurg 2007;106(3 Suppl): 196–200.

31. Tubbs RS, McGirt MJ, Oakes WJ. Surgical experience in 130 pediatric patients with CIMs. J Neurosurg 2003; 99:291–6.

Pathogenesis and Cerebrospinal Fluid Hydrodynamics of the Chiari I Malformation

Thomas J. Buell, MD[a], John D. Heiss, MD[b],
Edward H. Oldfield, MD[a],*

KEYWORDS

- Chiari I malformation • Hydrocephalus • Posterior fossa

KEY POINTS

- The pathogenesis of an anatomic Chiari I malformation can occur with several different mechanisms, including overcrowding from underdevelopment of the posterior fossa bony structures, hemodynamic disturbances of the central nervous system, such as hydrocephalus or bilateral chronic subdural hematomas producing tonsillar herniation, a mass in the posterior fossa causing tonsillar herniation, or, rarely, reduced spinal intrathecal pressure with downward herniation of the cerebellar tonsils associated with low spinal intrathecal pressure from a lumbar-to-peritoneal shunt or a spinal cerebrospinal fluid (CSF) leak.
- Because the abnormal shape and position of the cerebellar tonsils is reversed by surgery that provides unobstructed pulsatile movement of CSF across the foramen magnum, the pathogenesis of a Chiari I malformation is impaction of the tonsils in the foramen magnum, not a result of a congenital brain malformation.
- Evidence provided by anatomic imaging, dynamic imaging with MRI and intraoperative ultrasound, and physiologic studies during, before, and after surgery for Chiari I malformation is consistent with an extramedullary hydrodynamic mechanism in which the cerebellar tonsils are impacted in the foramen magnum and act on a partially entrapped spinal CSF space to increase intrathecal pressure and pulse pressure and produce suboccipital headache, and, in some patients, syringomyelia.
- Thus, the pathophysiology of the Chiari I malformation is simply the obstruction of the normal pulsatile movement of CSF across the foramen magnum.

INTRODUCTION

The pathology that is now known as Chiari malformations of the cerebellar tonsils originated in 1891 with Hans Chiari's manuscript titled "Concerning alterations in the cerebellum resulting from cerebral hydrocephalus."[1–3] In this publication, Chiari described "alterations in the cerebellum resulting from cerebral hydrocephalus."[1–3] In 1896, Chiari described an additional mechanism for the pathogenesis of the malformation; insufficient bone growth and insufficient enlargement of portions of

The authors report no financial conflicts of interest.

[a] Department of Neurological Surgery, University of Virginia Health System, P.O. Box 800212, Charlottesville, VA 22908, USA; [b] Surgical Neurology Branch, National Institutes of Health, 10 Center Drive, 10/3D20, MSC-1414, Bethesda, MD 20892, USA
* Corresponding author. Department of Neurological Surgery, University of Virginia Health System, P.O. Box 800212, Charlottesville, VA 22908, USA.
E-mail address: EHO4U@hscmail.mcc.virginia.edu

Neurosurg Clin N Am 26 (2015) 495–499
http://dx.doi.org/10.1016/j.nec.2015.06.003
1042-3680/15/$ – see front matter © 2015 Elsevier Inc. All rights reserved.

neurosurgery.theclinics.com

the skull during development cause increased intracranial pressure and subsequent tonsillar herniation.[3,4] Since Chiari's initial publications, there have been several hypotheses that attempt to elucidate the pathogenesis of the Chiari I malformation and the pathophysiology associated with it.

This article summarizes the current understanding of the pathophysiology of the Chiari malformation that is based on observations of the anatomy visualized by modern imaging with MRI and prospective studies of the physiology of patients before and after surgery. The pathogenesis of a Chiari I malformation of the cerebellar tonsils is grouped into 4 general mechanisms:

1. Overcrowding caused by underdevelopment of the posterior fossa bony structures
2. Hemodynamic disturbances that increase intracranial pressure
3. Excess tissue in the posterior fossa by a tumor
4. Downward movement of the central nervous system by events that lower intrathecal pressure, such as lumbar-to-peritoneal shunts.

It is noteworthy that each of these mechanisms acts on normal cerebellar tonsils to deform them by impacting them in the foramen magnum, deformation that is consistently reversed by simple surgery to provide extra room at the foramen magnum.

Of note, the authors have limited their comments to Type I Chiari malformation. Even with this limitation, it becomes apparent that unanimity of thought is lacking on the pathophysiology of the type I Chiari malformation. In fact, some hypotheses even contradict each other. For example, hydrocephalus has been proposed as both the etiologic cause and a result of the Chiari malformation.[5]

PATHOGENESIS OF THE CHIARI I MALFORMATION
Limited Embryologic Development of the Skull Base

Several studies have demonstrated that many, but not all, patients with a Chiari I have a small posterior fossa. In 1 study, to investigate overcrowding in the posterior cranial fossa as the pathogenesis of Chiari malformation, Nishikawa and colleagues[6] correlated the morphology of the brainstem and cerebellum with the anatomy of skull base. They used X-Ray tomography to measure 3 occipital enchondral parts: the supraocciput, exocciput, and basiocciput. They found a significant difference in the mean length of the exocciput, from the bottom of the occipital condyle to the top of the jugular tubercle, which measured 16 mm in

the Chiari group compared with 20.5 mm in control patients. They further described a significant difference in the length of the supraocciput between the internal occipital protuberance and the opisthion, which measured 38.9 mm in the Chiari group and 48.1 mm in the controls. The axial length of the clivus (the basiocciput and basisphenoid) in the Chiari group was not shorter than that of the control group. On average, the Chiari group had smaller posterior fossa cranial volume (186 cc) compared with the control group (193 cc), although it was not significant, and no significant difference was found in the posterior fossa brain volume (156 cc) compared with the controls (153 cc). As in other studies, there was a significant difference in the ratio of the posterior fossa brain volume to the posterior fossa cranial volume (mean volume ratio 0.833 in the Chiari group and 0.790 in the control group).[6]

Stovner and colleagues measured skull dimensions on lateral skull radiographs in 33 adult patients with MRI-verified Chiari malformations and 40 control subjects. They found that the posterior cranial fossa was significantly smaller and shallower in Chiari patients compared with controls. For Chiari patients, there was a positive correlation between posterior cranial fossa size and cerebellar tonsillar ectopia. Because of this positive correlation, Stovner and colleagues[7] propose that an undersized posterior cranial fossa had been expanded by hindbrain herniation at an early stage in development.

Vega and colleagues[8] studied a series of 42 patients with Chiari malformation compared with 46 control subjects. Their results support the hypothesis that cerebellar tonsillar ectopia is caused by the disproportionate size between the volume of the posterior cranial fossa and the cerebellum. The authors recorded linear, angular, and posterior fossa surface area measurements on lateral skull radiographs. They used computed tomography (CT) to calculate posterior cranial fossa volume. They found that Chiari patients exhibited shorter clival lengths, shorter Twining-opisthion distances, and shorter Chamberlain line. Also, the average size of the posterior cranial fossa was smaller in Chiari I patients compared with control.

Perhaps the most important and often ignored developmental feature that is related directly to the pathophysiology of Chiari malformation is the somatic origin of the occipital bone. Early in embryonic development, the occipital bone forms from at least 3 pairs of sclerotomes. The occipital sclerotomes, which in turn are formed from occipital somites, eventually fuse into a single structure and are incorporated into the developing cranial skeleton.[5] Marin-Padilla examined the hypothesis that primary para-axial mesodermal insufficiency (vitamin A-induced in their experimental model) can affect embryos after the closure of the neural folds and produce a Chiari I malformation. They found that mesodermal insufficiency can produce axial skeletal defects that prevent normal neural fold closure. They propose that the Chiari malformation may be secondary to primary mesodermal insufficiency during a particular embryonic stage in the closure of the neural folds. The authors tested this hypothesis with experimental models using vitamin A as a teratogen. They were able to induce the Chiari malformation in hamsters, which suggests that the condition can be caused by an error in posterior fossa development.[5]

Finally, as a result of animal breeding to produce the characteristic skull shape of King Charles Cavalier Spaniels several centuries ago, dogs were selected with a flat shape to the back of their heads. With the introduction of the use MRI in animals, this selective breeding for a small posterior fossa, was discovered to commonly be associated with Chiari I malformation and syringomyelia.[9]

The Chiari I malformation may be secondary to underdevelopment of the occipital enchondrium, possibly from underdevelopment of occipital somites. Overcrowding in the posterior cranial fossa, due to a normal-sized hindbrain in the presence of an underdeveloped occipital bone, causes cerebellar tonsillar ectopia. However, because only a portion of patients with a Chiari I malformation have a small posterior fossa, other factors can also produce a Chiari I abnormality of the cerebellar tonsils.[6]

Hemodynamic Disturbance of the Central Nervous System

At the Cleveland Clinic in the 1950s, James Gardner, in a series of reports, established that the Chiari I malformation was the most common cause of syringomyelia.[10] He proposed that the fundamental mechanism underlying the origin of the Chiari malformation is delayed opening of the membrane covering the outlet of the fourth ventricle during fetal development and transient obstructive hydrocephalus with resulting foraminal herniation of the hindbrain and cerebellar tonsils. One of the difficulties with this potential mechanism is that it would not explain the small posterior fossa that has been described by several investigators in many patients with a Chiari I malformation since Gardner's reports.[10]

The experimental observations of Margolis and Kilham with the reovirus-induced hydrocephalus are of considerable interest for the understanding of the morphogenesis of Chiari malformation. They inoculated hamsters postnatally with type I reovirus. This virus selectively destroys the ventricular ependymal layer, causing an inflammatory response with subsequent gliosis. The result is an obliteration of the ventricular system at strategic points, such as the aqueduct of Sylvius, producing rapid hydrocephalus followed by cerebellar herniation. The authors propose that the Chiari malformation is caused by 2 factors:

1. The rapidly growing hydrocephalic brain will occupy the entire cranial vault including the posterior cranial fossa.
2. Due to the reduced available space in the posterior cranial fossa, the cerebellum is forced to herniate into the cervical canal, because the entire cranial vault is already filled to maximal capacity.[5,11]

In the clinic, the Chiari I malformation has also been shown to be a result of hydrocephalus and with bilateral supratentorial chronic subdural hematomas with complete resolution of the Chiari I abnormality after successful treatment.[12–14]

Herniation of the Cerebellar Tonsils Associated with Posterior Fossa Tumors

It has long been known that the mass effect of a posterior fossa tumor can produce herniation of the cerebellar tonsils with a shape that is identical to the shape of the tonsils associated with idiopathic Chiari I malformation. In 1 study, tonsil herniation identical to Chiari I malformation was evident on MRI in 24 of 164 patients with posterior fossa tumors, at least five of whom also had syringomyelia.[15]

Cranio-Spinal Pressure Imbalance Associated with Low Spinal Intrathecal Pressure

Reduced spinal intrathecal pressure with downward herniation of the cerebellar tonsils as a result of a cranio-spinal pressure imbalance caused by low spinal intrathecal pressure from a lumbar-to-peritoneal shunt or a spinal CSF leak has been known since shortly after the introduction of lumbar-to-peritoneal shunting procedures, and its presence is now considered the rule, rather than the exception, with lumbar-to-peritoneal shunting.[16,17]

Complete Reversal of the Abnormal Shape and Position of the Chiari I Malformation with Surgical Treatment of Syringomyelia

The conclusion that the typical abnormal shape and position of the cerebellar tonsils is acquired, rather than congenital, is clearly shown by complete reversion to a normal position and shape of the cerebellar tonsils in the months after successful surgery.[18]

PATHOPHYSIOLOGY ASSOCIATED WITH CHIARI I MALFORMATION

Prospective studies to examine the pathophysiology of Chiari I malformation were performed at the National Institute of Health (NIH). The NIH studies used techniques to assess anatomy, physiology with direct pressure measurements, and dynamic imaging of the tonsils with MRI and intraoperative ultrasound. This permitted simultaneous assessment and correlation of anatomic changes during the cardiac cycle with abnormal pressures. The findings of those studies have been detailed in a series of publications.[19–21] The findings of the abnormal pathophysiology have been consistent over the course of several studies, including patients with syringomyelia caused by a Chiari I malformation, patients with persistent or recurrent syringomyelia after unsuccessful surgery, and patients with primary spinal syringomyelia.[22]

Those studies indicate that a Chiari I malformation partially obstructs the free movement of CSF across the foramen magnum. In normal subjects, it is known that as cardiac systole rapidly delivers blood to the brain, the capacitance of the venous system of the brain absorbs much of the new volume of blood arriving at the intracranial space. However, during systole, about 0.75 to 1.0 mL of CSF are also rapidly moved from the cisterna magna across the subarachnoid space and into the spinal subarachnoid space at the level of the foramen magnum. That extra amount of CSF that is now in the spinal intrathecal system then moves back to the cranial space during diastole.

With a Chiari I malformation, the tonsils are impacted into the foramen magnum, blocking the rapid movement of CSF that normally occurs across that space during systole. That occlusion partially entraps the spinal intrathecal space, resulting in reduced compliance in the spinal CSF space. Now, rather than the CSF moving in and out of the head during the cardiac cycle, the tonsils rapidly move downward to provide accommodation that would normally be provided by the CSF, leaving the head and moving into the spine. That tonsil movement is against a partially entrapped CSF space with reduced compliance. In this abnormal circumstance, the tonsils act as a piston on the partially entrapped spinal CSF space to produce increased intrathecal pressure and increased pulse pressure. All these features of pathophysiology were established in the series of prospective clinical studies of Chiari I malformation at the NIH in patients with Chiari I malformation, with or without syringomyelia.[19–21]

SUMMARY

It is clear from many lines of evidence and from a broad spectrum of different circumstances that the abnormal shape of the cerebellar tonsils with a Chiari I malformation is simply a shape that is imposed on the tonsils by their impaction in the foramen magnum. This impaction occurs during the systolic delivery of blood to the brain, which occurs 100,000 to 120,000 times each day. Thus, any process that produces tonsil herniation through the foramen magnum, whether it is a small posterior fossa, herniation produced by hydrocephalous or a posterior fossa tumor, or low intrathecal CSF pressure, has the potential of producing the anatomic abnormality that is commonly called a Chiari I abnormality. The pathophysiology resulting from that impaction is simply obstruction of the free pulsatile movement of CSF across the foramen magnum, which produces the suboccipital headaches that patients experience, as well as the cough headaches and the pathophysiology underlying syringomyelia affecting some patients.

REFERENCES

1. Chiari H. Über Veranderungen des Kleinhirns in Folge von Hydrocephalie des Grosshirns. Dtsch Med Wschr 1891;17:1171–5.
2. John A, Anson EC, Issam AA. Syringomyelia and the chiari malformations. Neurosurgical topics. AANS Publications Committee. J Bone Joint Surg Am 1997;80(2):308.
3. Bejjani GK. Definition of the adult Chiari malformation: a brief historical overview. Neurosurg Focus 2001;11(1):E1.
4. Chiari H. Uber die Veranderungen des Kleinhirns, der Pons under Medulla oblongata in Folge von congenitaler Hydrocephalie des Grosshirns. Denkschr Akad Wiss Wien 1896;63:71–116.
5. Marin-Padilla M, Marin-Padilla TM. Morphogenesis of experimentally induced Arnold–Chiari malformation. J Neurol Sci 1981;50(1):29–55.
6. Nishikawa M, Sakamoto H, Hakuba A, et al. Pathogenesis of Chiari malformation: a morphometric study of the posterior cranial fossa. J Neurosurg 1997;86(1):40–7.
7. Stovner LJ, Bergan U, Nilsen G, et al. Posterior cranial fossa dimensions in the Chiari I malformation: relation to pathogenesis and clinical presentation. Neuroradiology 1993;35(2):113–8.

8. Vega A, Quintana F, Berciano J. Basichondrocranium anomalies in adult Chiari type I malformation: a morphometric study. J Neurol Sci 1990;99(2–3): 137–45.

9. Rusbridge C, Knowler SP. Inheritance of occipital bone hypoplasia (Chiari Type I Malformation) in Cavalier King Charles Spaniels. J Vet Intern Med 2004;18:673–8.

10. Gardner WJ, Goodall RJ. The surgical treatment of Arnold-Chiari malformation in adults; an explanation of its mechanism and importance of encephalography in diagnosis. J Neurosurg 1950;7(3):199–206.

11. Margolis G, Kilham L. Experimental virus-induced hydrocephalus. Relation to pathogenesis of the Arnold-Chiari malformation. J Neurosurg 1969; 31(1):1–9.

12. Di Rocco C, Frassanito P, Massimi L, et al. Hydrocephalus and Chiari type I malformation. Childs Nerv Syst 2011;27(10):1653–64.

13. Morioka T, Shono T, Nishio S, et al. Acquired Chiari I malformation and syringomyelia associated with bilateral chronic subdural hematoma. Case report. J Neurosurg 1995;83(3):556–8.

14. Wen L, Ma C, Wang H, et al. The role of hydrocephalus in the development of Chiari I malformation and syringomyelia. J Neurol Sci 2014;344(1–2):240–2.

15. Tachibana S, Harada K, Abe T, et al. Syringomyelia secondary to tonsillar herniation caused by posterior fossa tumors. Surg Neurol 1995;43(5):470–5 [discussion: 475–7].

16. Welch K, Shillito J, Strand R, et al. Chiari I "malformations"—an acquired disorder? J Neurosurg 1981;55(4):604–9.

17. Chumas PD, Armstrong DC, Drake JM, et al. Tonsillar herniation: the rule rather than the exception after lumboperitoneal shunting in the pediatric population. J Neurosurg 1993;78(4):568–73.

18. Heiss JD, Suffredini G, Bakhtian KD, et al. Normalization of hindbrain morphology after decompression of Chiari malformation Type I. J Neurosurg 2012; 117(5):942–6.

19. Heiss J, Suffredini G, Smith R. Comment: pathophysiology of persistent syringomyelia after decompressive craniocervical surgery. Clinical article. J Neurosurg Spine 2010;13(6):729–42.

20. Heiss JD, Patronas N, DeVroom HL, et al. Elucidating the pathophysiology of syringomyelia. J Neurosurg 1999;91(4):553–62.

21. Oldfield EH, Muraszko K, Shawker TH, et al. Pathophysiology of syringomyelia associated with Chiari I malformation of the cerebellar tonsils. Implications for diagnosis and treatment. J Neurosurg 1994; 80(1):3–15.

22. Heiss JD, Snyder K, Peterson MM, et al. Pathophysiology of primary spinal syringomyelia. J Neurosurg Spine 2012;17(5):367–80.

Prevalence of Chiari I Malformation and Syringomyelia

Elyne N. Kahn, MD, Karin M. Muraszko, MD,
Cormac O. Maher, MD*

KEYWORDS

• Chiari • Prevalence • Incidence • Syrinx • Imaging

KEY POINTS

• Defining prevalence of Chiari I malformation is challenging. Existing studies are limited by detection bias.
• Asymptomatic Chiari I malformation is common.
• Symptomatic Chiari I malformation is less common.
• Prevalence of Chiari I malformation likely decreases with older age.
• Spinal cord syrinx in the context of Chiari I malformation tends to occur in the cervical spinal cord and is increasingly seen with progressively lower tonsil position.

IMAGING PREVALENCE OF CHIARI I MALFORMATION

Chiari I malformation (CM) is a common neurosurgical diagnosis and spinal cord syrinx is frequently found in patients with CM.[1–10] However, it has been difficult to establish the true prevalence of these two associated conditions. Determining the population prevalence of CM and any associated spinal syringes would require evaluating every individual within a population of interest using a tool that is both perfectly sensitive and perfectly specific for this condition. Because such a study has so far proved to be impossible, clinicians must rely on imperfect estimates of CM and syrinx prevalence. The largest studies of CM prevalence retrospectively reviewed large numbers of patients selected for brain and spine imaging. Rather than defining the true population prevalence, these studies describe, by definition, the imaging prevalence of the condition.[11–15]

The main limitation of this approach is that individuals undergoing MRI are not representative of the general population. Because patients with neurologic symptoms are more likely to undergo neuroimaging, imaging prevalence estimates are influenced by detection bias when the condition is associated with symptoms. Conditions that are usually symptomatic are over-represented in imaging prevalence studies because of detection bias. For this reason, imaging prevalence estimates are expected to correlate more precisely with true population prevalence estimates for asymptomatic conditions compared with symptomatic diseases. Their limitations notwithstanding, these imaging prevalence studies have provided the best estimates of CM prevalence in the population, especially given the large numbers of asymptomatic individuals who meet imaging criteria for the diagnosis. In addition, they provide insight into the prevalence of spinal cord syrinx in the context of CM.

Disclosures: The authors have no conflicts of interest to disclose.
Department of Neurosurgery, University of Michigan, Ann Arbor, MI, USA
* Corresponding author. Department of Neurosurgery, University of Michigan, 1500 East Medical Center Drive, Room 3552 TC, Ann Arbor, MI 48109-5338.
E-mail address: cmaher@med.umich.edu

On imaging, CM is typically defined by cerebellar tonsil position 5 mm or more below the foramen magnum.[15–18] Using this definition, imaging prevalence studies estimate CM prevalence at between 0.24% and 3.6% of the population.[11–15] Variation in these estimates may be attributed to differences in sensitivity of CM detection between studies as well as differences in the populations being analyzed. For instance, some studies have focused exclusively on children,[11,14] others exclusively on adults,[15] and others on both children and adults.[12] For CM, the age of the population being examined significantly influences prevalence estimates. In a retrospective review of 22,591 patients undergoing brain MRI at a single institution, Meadows and colleagues[12] found that 175 patients (0.77%) met imaging criteria for CM. These investigators did not report age-specific or age group–specific prevalence. Strahle and colleagues[14] focused on the pediatric population in a retrospective review of 14,116 consecutive patients aged 18 years or younger who had undergone brain or cervical spine MRI at a single institution. They identified 509 patients with CM, representing 3.6% of the imaged population. The discrepancy between these estimates is a result of the different age groups analyzed. The prevalence of low tonsil position as well as CM on MRI is substantially higher in children and young adults compared with older adults.[19,20] Any study that includes a large number of older adults will find a lower prevalence compared with an analysis focused on children.

Although no lifelong natural history studies have been performed, the changes in age-specific imaging prevalence probably reflect changes that occur in individuals during their lifetimes. Tonsil position should not be expected to be static over the course of a lifetime. Several investigators have reported spontaneous resolution of childhood CM and associated syringes.[21,22] Mikulis and colleagues[19] were the first investigators to analyze and report on age-related changes in normal cerebellar tonsil position. They identified a trend toward more cranial tonsil position with increasing age. However, their analysis was limited by a small sample size. More recently, Smith and colleagues[20] measured cerebellar tonsil position in a large number of patients who had undergone MRI for any reason, and they compared tonsil positions according to age (**Fig. 1**). Mean cerebellar tonsil position descended with advancing age into young adulthood, then ascended with advancing age throughout adult life. In all age groups studied, cerebellar tonsil position follows a normal or near-normal distribution (**Fig. 2**). Individuals with tonsil position at the low end of this distribution are within the group that is usually considered consistent with an imaging diagnosis of CM. This finding has implications for disease nosology as it relates to CM. Individuals with this imaging finding are at the low end of a continuous spectrum of tonsil positions found in humans. Female sex is associated with a higher prevalence of CM on imaging.[12,14,23,24] Female patients seem to have lower cerebellar tonsil positions compared with male patients in all age groups.[20] Obesity or increased body mass index does not seem to be related to the prevalence of CM on imaging.[25]

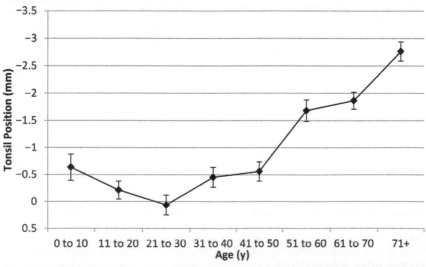

Fig. 1. Mean lowest tonsil position by age in 2400 patients undergoing imaging. (*From* Smith BW, Strahle J, Bapuraj JR, et al. Distribution of cerebellar tonsil position: implications for understanding Chiari malformation. J Neurosurg 2013;119(3):816; with permission.)

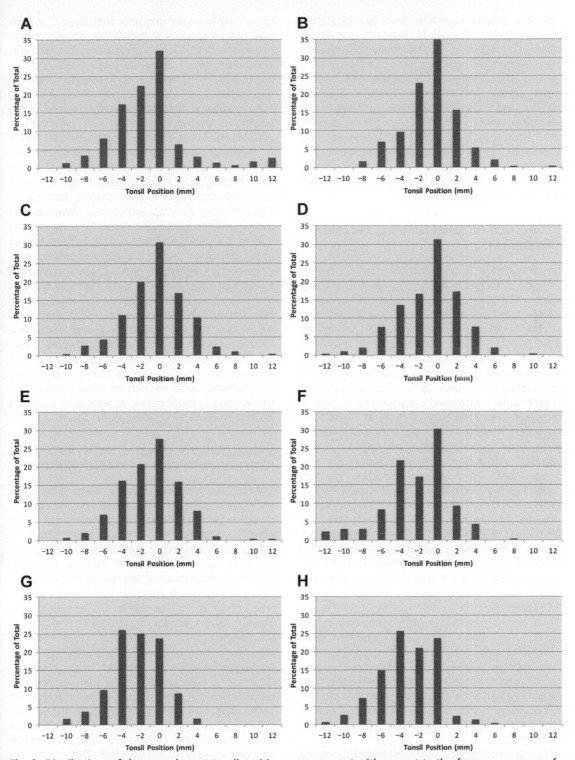

Fig. 2. Distributions of the mean lowest tonsil position measurement with respect to the foramen magnum for the following age groups: 0 to 10 years (*A*), 11 to 20 years (*B*), 21 to 30 years (*C*), 31 to 40 years (*D*), 41 to 50 years (*E*), 51 to 60 years (*F*), 61 to 70 years (*G*), and 71 years or older (*H*). Negative numbers correspond with a more rostral tonsil location with respect to the foramen magnum. (*From* Smith BW, Strahle J, Bapuraj JR, et al. Distribution of cerebellar tonsil position: implications for understanding Chiari malformation. J Neurosurg 2013;119(3):817; with permission.)

Several groups have attempted to mitigate the detection bias inherent in imaging prevalence analyses by reporting on intracranial findings after MRI screening of healthy adult volunteers.[15,26–28] Vernooij and colleagues[15] screened 2000 healthy adults more than 45 years of age. Eighteen (0.9%) of the volunteers had CM. Each study that relies on volunteers is subject to negative selection bias, because individuals with symptoms are likely to be excluded. As well as specific age criteria, this limits reliable extrapolation of results to the general population. None of these studies of healthy volunteers have included children.

PREVALENCE OF SYMPTOMATIC CHIARI I MALFORMATION

The prevalence of symptomatic CM is distinct from the population prevalence of anatomically defined CM on imaging. Symptomatic cases of CM seem to have a very low incidence compared with any of the recent estimates for CM prevalence as an imaging finding, which suggests that most cases of CM found incidentally on imaging are asymptomatic. In the series reported by Strahle and colleagues,[14] only 32% of cases detected on MRI were considered symptomatic at time of diagnosis. Given the large number of asymptomatic cases, there are many patients who likely will never come to medical attention. Aitken and colleagues[11] also found a low prevalence of symptomatic CM. They studied pediatric patients enrolled in the Northern California Kaiser Permanente system in 1997 and 1998.[11] The population consisted of a total of 741,815 patients less than 20 years of age. Within the 2-year study period, 5248 (0.71%) of those patients underwent MRI of the head or spine. CM was identified in 51 patients, representing a 2-year period prevalence of 1.0% in the imaged population. The frequency of CM diagnoses in the total population, reflecting a 2-year period prevalence of symptomatic cases, was 0.7 per 10,000 (0.007%). Furthermore, even in patients who are symptomatic, diagnosis is often delayed. Aitken and colleagues[11] noted that, among symptomatic patients with CM in their study, only half were diagnosed within 14 months of symptom onset, and a quarter of patients were diagnosed only after a period greater than 106 months.

Several investigators have identified associations for symptomatic rather than asymptomatic CM on imaging. Some, but not all, studies have found that lower tonsil position and more severe alterations in cerebrospinal fluid (CSF) flow at the foramen magnum are significantly associated with a higher likelihood of symptoms.[11,14] Girls are more likely to be symptomatic than boys.[14] In general, patient age has a remarkable correlation between most frequent symptomatic presentation and lowest mean cerebellar tonsil position in the population.[20] In pediatric populations, symptomatic patients are likely to be older.[11,18,24,29,30] Mean cerebellar tonsil position ascends throughout adulthood, perhaps explaining why symptomatic presentation in the elderly is much less common.[20]

Several groups have examined the natural history of asymptomatic or minimally symptomatic CM on imaging in order to determine how often asymptomatic patients with imaging findings of CM ultimately develop symptoms. Novegno and colleagues[24] followed 22 patients for a mean duration of 5.9 years and found that 5 patients had some clinical worsening. Benglis and colleagues[31] followed 124 patients over a 2.8-year interval and found that most patients were clinically beyond that interval. In addition, Strahle and colleagues[32] followed 147 patients over a mean interval of 4.6 years and found that 9 patients had new symptoms possibly related to the CM during that interval. Taken together, these studies suggest that the natural history of asymptomatic or minimally symptomatic patients with imaging evidence of CM is good in most cases, at least over the short intervals reported in the literature.

PREVALENCE OF SPINAL CORD SYRINX IN PATIENTS WITH CHIARI I MALFORMATION

CM is known to be associated with spinal cord syrinx in many patients.[1–10] Studies of patients undergoing surgery have reported a prevalence of spinal syrinx in 60% to 85% of patients with CM.[33–35] Presence of a syrinx is considered by many surgeons to be an indication for surgery; however, these reports probably overestimate the frequency of syrinx in patients with CM.[36–38] The true prevalence of syrinx in this population remains poorly defined. Some insight is provided by studies of the imaging prevalence of CM, which have attempted to define the imaging prevalence of syrinx among those patients with CM. In the study by Strahle and colleagues,[14] most patients had undergone MRI of the cervical spine to screen for syrinx, half had undergone imaging of the total spine, and 22.9% of patients with CM also had a syrinx. Aitken and colleagues[11] identified spinal syringes in 12% of patients with CM. It may be that screening methods used in this study were less sensitive in detecting syrinx. It is also possible that these imaging studies overestimated the prevalence of syrinx in children with CM, given that the children who were referred for spine imaging may have an increased likelihood of syrinx

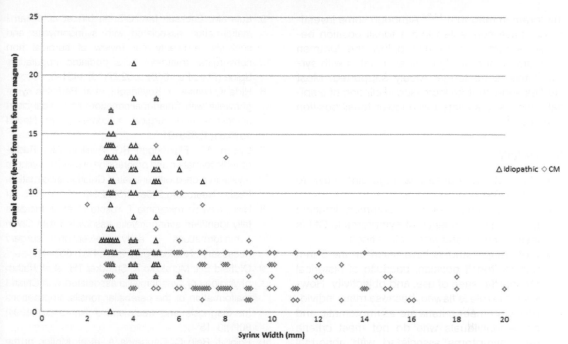

Fig. 3. Patients with idiopathic and CM-associated syrinx grouped according to maximum syrinx width and cranial extent of syrinx. (*From* Strahle J, Muraszko KM, Garton HJ, et al. Syrinx location and size according to etiology: identification of Chiari-associated syrinx. J Neurosurg Pediatr 2015;16(1):25; with permission.)

compared with those children with CM who were not referred for spine imaging.

CM-associated syringes tend to occur in the cervical spinal cord (**Fig. 3**).[11,14,39] Characteristics associated with a higher prevalence of syrinx include female sex, older age, pegged (as opposed to rounded) tonsil shape, basilar invagination, and greater mean tonsillar descent below

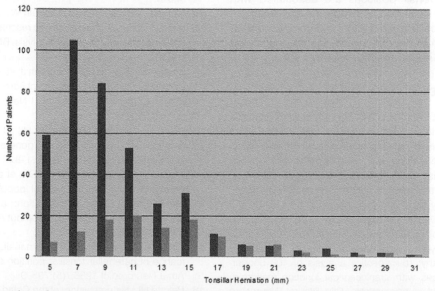

Fig. 4. The number of patients with CM alone (black bars) versus those with both CM and syrinx (gray bars), according to the measurement (in millimeters) of tonsillar descent below the foramen magnum. Patients with greater amounts of tonsillar decent were more likely to have an associated syrinx. (*From* Strahle J, Muraszko KM, Kapurch J, et al. Chiari malformation type I and syrinx in children undergoing magnetic resonance imaging. J Neurosurg Pediatr 2011;8(2):208; with permission.)

the foramen magnum.[14,39] Although some investigators have suggested that a tonsil position between 9 mm and 14 mm below the foramen magnum is more likely to be associated with syrinx,[40] this is no longer widely supported. Most studies show that an increased likelihood of a spinal syrinx is associated with lower tonsil position **(Fig. 4)**.[14,23,41]

SUMMARY

- There is no consensus regarding how to define CM.
- Asymptomatic CM is a common imaging finding. The incidence of symptomatic CM is less common and also well defined.
- Most major studies have relied on the 5-mm rule for tonsil position, because of historical standards, ease of use, and objectivity. However, the rule is flawed, because many individuals who meet criteria are asymptomatic and some individuals who do not meet criteria have symptoms associated with abnormal CSF flow and crowding of structures at the foramen magnum.
- We think that the 5-mm rule for tonsil position should not be considered a definitive threshold with definite pathologic consequences. A tonsil position 5 mm or more below the foramen magnum is the low end of a continuous population distribution that results in a clinical syndrome in some individuals.
- Lower tonsil positions are associated with greater likelihood of symptoms and syrinx.
- Evidence suggests that the natural history for asymptomatic or minimally symptomatic individuals is good in most cases.

REFERENCES

1. Armonda RA, Citrin CM, Foley KT, et al. Quantitative cine-mode magnetic resonance imaging of Chiari I malformations: an analysis of cerebrospinal fluid dynamics. Neurosurgery 1994;35(2):214–24.
2. Blagodatsky MD, Larionov SN, Manohin PA, et al. Surgical treatment of "hindbrain related" syringomyelia: new data for pathogenesis. Acta Neurochir (Wien) 1993;124(2–4):82–5.
3. Bogdanov EI, Mendelevich EG. Syrinx size and duration of symptoms predict the pace of progressive myelopathy: retrospective analysis of 103 unoperated cases with craniocervical junction malformations and syringomyelia. Clin Neurol Neurosurg 2002;104(2):90–7.
4. Cahan LD, Bentson JR. Considerations in the diagnosis and treatment of syringomyelia and the Chiari malformation. J Neurosurg 1982;57(1):24–31.
5. Eule JM, Erickson MA, O'Brien MF, et al. Chiari I malformation associated with syringomyelia and scoliosis: a twenty-year review of surgical and nonsurgical treatment in a pediatric population. Spine (Phila Pa 1976) 2002;27(13):1451–5.
6. Hida K, Iwasaki Y, Koyanagi I, et al. Pediatric syringomyelia with Chiari malformation: its clinical characteristics and surgical outcomes. Surg Neurol 1999;51(4):383–91.
7. Lipson AC, Ellenbogen RG, Avellino AM. Radiographic formation and progression of cervical syringomyelia in a child with untreated Chiari I malformation. Pediatr Neurosurg 2008;44(3):221–3.
8. Nishizawa S, Yokoyama T, Yokota N, et al. Incidentally identified syringomyelia associated with Chiari I malformations: is early interventional surgery necessary? Neurosurgery 2001;49(3):637–41.
9. Oldfield EH, Muraszko K, Shawker TH, et al. Pathophysiology of syringomyelia associated with Chiari I malformation of the cerebellar tonsils. Implications for diagnosis and treatment. J Neurosurg 1994;80(1):3–15.
10. Pujol J, Roig C, Capdevila A, et al. Motion of the cerebellar tonsils in Chiari type I malformation studied by cine phase-contrast MRI. Neurology 1995;45(9):1746–53.
11. Aitken LA, Lindan CE, Sidney S, et al. Chiari type I malformation in a pediatric population. Pediatr Neurol 2009;40(6):449–54.
12. Meadows J, Kraut M, Guarnieri M, et al. Asymptomatic Chiari Type I malformations identified on magnetic resonance imaging. J Neurosurg 2000;92(6):920–6.
13. Morris Z, Whiteley WN, Longstreth WT Jr, et al. Incidental findings on brain magnetic resonance imaging: systematic review and meta-analysis. BMJ 2009;339:b3016.
14. Strahle J, Muraszko KM, Kapurch J, et al. Chiari malformation Type I and syrinx in children undergoing magnetic resonance imaging. J Neurosurg Pediatr 2011;8(2):205–13.
15. Vernooij MW, Ikram MA, Tanghe HL, et al. Incidental findings on brain MRI in the general population. N Engl J Med 2007;357(18):1821–8.
16. Aboulezz AO, Sartor K, Geyer CA, et al. Position of cerebellar tonsils in the normal population and in patients with Chiari malformation: a quantitative approach with MR imaging. J Comput Assist Tomogr 1985;9(6):1033–6.
17. Barkovich AJ, Wippold FJ, Sherman JL, et al. Significance of cerebellar tonsillar position on MR. AJNR Am J Neuroradiol 1986;7(5):795–9.
18. Rekate HL. Natural history of the Chiari Type I anomaly. J Neurosurg Pediatr 2008;2(3):177–8.
19. Mikulis DJ, Diaz O, Egglin TK, et al. Variance of the position of the cerebellar tonsils with age: preliminary report. Radiology 1992;183(3):725–8.

20. Smith BW, Strahle J, Bapuraj JR, et al. Distribution of cerebellar tonsil position: implications for understanding Chiari malformation. J Neurosurg 2013; 119(3):812–9.

21. Avellino AM, Britz GW, McDowell JR, et al. Spontaneous resolution of a cervicothoracic syrinx in a child. Case report and review of the literature. Pediatr Neurosurg 1999;30(1):43–6.

22. Sun PP, Harrop J, Sutton LN, et al. Complete spontaneous resolution of childhood Chiari I malformation and associated syringomyelia. Pediatrics 2001; 107(1):182–4.

23. Elster AD, Chen MY. Chiari I malformations: clinical and radiologic reappraisal. Radiology 1992;183(2): 347–53.

24. Novegno F, Caldarelli M, Massa A, et al. The natural history of the Chiari Type I anomaly. J Neurosurg Pediatr 2008;2(3):179–87.

25. Smith BW, Strahle J, Kazarian E, et al. Impact of body mass index on cerebellar tonsil position in healthy subjects and patients with Chiari malformation. J Neurosurg 2015;3:1–6.

26. Katzman GL, Dagher AP, Patronas NJ. Incidental findings on brain magnetic resonance imaging from 1000 asymptomatic volunteers. JAMA 1999; 282(1):36–9.

27. Weber F, Knopf H. Cranial MRI as a screening tool: findings in 1,772 military pilot applicants. Aviat Space Environ Med 2004;75(2):158–61.

28. Yue NC, Longstreth WT Jr, Elster AD, et al. Clinically serious abnormalities found incidentally at MR imaging of the brain: data from the Cardiovascular Health Study. Radiology 1997;202(1):41–6.

29. Genitori L, Peretta P, Nurisso C, et al. Chiari type I anomalies in children and adolescents: minimally invasive management in a series of 53 cases. Childs Nerv Syst 2000;16(10–11):707–18.

30. Navarro R, Olavarria G, Seshadri R, et al. Surgical results of posterior fossa decompression for patients with Chiari I malformation. Childs Nerv Syst 2004; 20(5):349–56.

31. Benglis D Jr, Covington D, Bhatia R, et al. Outcomes in pediatric patients with Chiari malformation Type I followed up without surgery. J Neurosurg Pediatr 2011;7(4):375–9.

32. Strahle J, Muraszko KM, Kapurch J, et al. Natural history of Chiari malformation Type I following decision for conservative treatment. J Neurosurg Pediatr 2011;8(2):214–21.

33. Tubbs RS, Webb DB, Oakes WJ. Persistent syringomyelia following pediatric Chiari I decompression: radiological and surgical findings. J Neurosurg 2004;100(5 Suppl Pediatrics):460–4.

34. Menezes AH. Chiari I malformations and hydromyelia–complications. Pediatr Neurosurg 1991;17(3): 146–54.

35. Milhorat TH, Chou MW, Trinidad EM, et al. Chiari I malformation redefined: clinical and radiographic findings for 364 symptomatic patients. Neurosurgery 1999;44(5):1005–17.

36. Haines SJ, Berger M. Current treatment of Chiari malformations types I and II: A survey of the Pediatric Section of the American Association of Neurological Surgeons. Neurosurgery 1991;28(3):353–7.

37. Haroun RI, Guarnieri M, Meadow JJ, et al. Current opinions for the treatment of syringomyelia and Chiari malformations: survey of the Pediatric Section of the American Association of Neurological Surgeons. Pediatr Neurosurg 2000;33(6):311–7.

38. Schijman E, Steinbok P. International survey on the management of Chiari I malformation and syringomyelia. Childs Nerv Syst 2004;20(5):341–8.

39. Strahle J, Muraszko KM, Garton HJ, et al. Syrinx location and size according to etiology: identification of Chiari-associated syrinx. J Neurosurg Pediatr 2015;3:1–9.

40. Stovner LJ, Rinck P. Syringomyelia in Chiari malformation: relation to extent of cerebellar tissue herniation. Neurosurgery 1992;31(5):913–7.

41. Pillay PK, Awad IA, Little JR, et al. Symptomatic Chiari malformation in adults: a new classification based on magnetic resonance imaging with clinical and prognostic significance. Neurosurgery 1991; 28(5):639–45.

Clinical Presentation of Chiari I Malformation and Syringomyelia in Children

Jonathan Pindrik, MD, James M. Johnston Jr, MD*

KEYWORDS

- Chiari I malformation • Syringomyelia • Syrinx • Scoliosis • Headache • Cervicomedullary junction
- Craniocervical junction

KEY POINTS

- Chiari I malformation (CM1) may present with varying symptoms depending on patient age, or may represent an incidental finding in asymptomatic patients.
- The most common clinical presentations of CM1 in children involve occipital headache or posterior cervical pain, syringomyelia, and/or scoliosis.
- The constellation of symptoms and signs in CM1 relate to brainstem or cervical spinal cord compression, lower cranial nerve dysfunction, and/or syringomyelia.
- Clinical examination signs in children with CM1 may include sensorimotor deficits, lower cranial nerve deficits, or signs of medullary dysfunction.
- In rare circumstances, children with CM1 may present with acute onset or rapidly progressive findings warranting urgent surgical consideration.

INTRODUCTION

Chiari I malformation (CM1) refers to abnormal cerebellar tonsillar descent below the foramen magnum, typically at least 5 mm below this level for a qualifying diagnosis.[1–6] This form of hindbrain herniation may present with commonly recognized or rarely reported clinical symptoms, and also may be found incidentally. The frequency of radiographic findings consistent with CM1 among children undergoing brain and/or spine imaging for any indication has been estimated to be as high as 3% to 4%.[7] Symptoms from CM1 generally exhibit the following characteristics[7]:

- Clinical presentation (symptoms, signs) vary with respect to age; and
- Younger patients tend to present sooner, with shorter symptom duration, than adult patients.

As described more thoroughly in this article, tonsillar impaction within the foramen magnum causes compression of the cervicomedullary junction. The resulting compression and abnormal cerebrospinal fluid flow dynamics across the craniocervical junction result in a differential pressure gradient.[1–3,5,6,8,9] Thus, the clinical presentation of CM1 in children may reflect a constellation of symptoms resulting from compression at the cervicomedullary junction and those related to syringomyelia and scoliosis.[7,10,11] However, as with many neurosurgical conditions based partly on radiographic findings, CM1 may be discovered

Disclosures: The authors have no commercial or financial conflicts of interest to report. There were no funding sources for the completion of this work.
Division of Pediatric Neurosurgery, Department of Neurosurgery, Children's of Alabama, University of Alabama, Birmingham (UAB), 1600 7th Avenue South, Lowder 400, Birmingham, AL 35233, USA
* Corresponding author.
E-mail address: James.Johnston@childrensal.org

Neurosurg Clin N Am 26 (2015) 509–514
http://dx.doi.org/10.1016/j.nec.2015.06.004
1042-3680/15/$ – see front matter © 2015 Elsevier Inc. All rights reserved.

incidentally within asymptomatic patients or patients evaluated for nonspecific symptoms like headache or dizziness. Approximately 15% to 37% of pediatric patients with radiographic evidence of inferior cerebellar tonsillar ectopia may be asymptomatic, based on large retrospective reviews.[4,12,13] Additionally, patients may develop acquired tonsillar descent owing to other causes (posterior fossa mass, lumbar cerebrospinal fluid drainage/leakage, etc).

The most common clinical presentations of CM1 involve headaches and/or neck pain and scoliosis (most commonly levoscoliosis; **Table 1**).[2,4,7,8,12,14] Headaches represent a significant component of the clinical presentation in 27% to 70% of children with symptomatic CM1.[2,3,5,7,12,15] Classically, headaches in adolescents and adults demonstrate an occipitocervical location and are provoked or intensified by Valsalva-type maneuvers, with relatively ephemeral duration.[1,2,4–8,10,12,14] Various functions or activities that induce a Valsalva-type response, consistent with childhood behavior, include[7]:

- Sneezing, coughing;
- Laughing, screaming;
- Defecation; and
- Running, repetitive jumping.

Younger patients (neonates, infants, toddlers) often may fail to demonstrate or adequately communicate these classic headache descriptors.[12]

Characterized objectively by Cobb angles, scoliosis demonstrates strong association with syringomyelia in CM1.[6–9,14] In general, the following rules apply[2,8,9]:

- Most (but not all) pediatric CM1 patients with scoliosis have underlying syringomyelia; and
- Not all CM1 patients with syringomyelia have scoliosis.

Syringomyelia in CM1 demonstrates predilection for the following regions[2,3]:

- Cervical spinal cord (15%–21%),
- Cervicothoracic spinal cord (12%–25%);
- Thoracic spinal cord (15%–16%);

Table 1
Common clinical presentations of Chiari I malformation and syringomyelia in children

Clinical Sign or Symptom	Reported Prevalence in Pediatric CM1 Population[a]
Headache, neck pain	27%–70%
Scoliosis	18%–50%
Motor or sensory deficits of the extremities Paresis (typically in the upper extremities) Sensory deficits (in upper and/or lower extremities) Decrement of fine motor control	6%–17%
Irritability (typically younger patients)	12%
Oropharyngeal dysfunction, dysphagia, dysarthria Absent or reduced gag reflex Decreased palatal elevation Vocal cord dysfunction, hoarseness Tongue atrophy	4%–15%
Sleep apnea or bradycardia	4%–13%
Spasticity, hyperreflexia (typically in the lower extremities) Reflection of upper motor neuron impairment	6%
Frequent emesis	1%–10%
Ataxia or gait impairment, decreased coordination	4%–9%
Dysesthetic pain in C2 dermatomal distribution	7%
Facial numbness (trigeminal nerve sensory deficits)	7%
Auditory symptoms (tinnitus, hearing loss)	2%
Respiratory difficulty, dyspnea, stridor	1%–2%
Atrophy, hyporeflexia, and/or fasciculations in upper extremities Reflection of lower motor neuron impairment	Not reported

[a] Prevalence estimates are based on frequencies reported in peer-reviewed publications, and likely represent upper estimates in most cases.
Data from Refs.[2–4,7,8,10–12,14,15,17]

- Lumbar spinal cord (3%–4%); and
- Holocord (39%–44%).

Less common but concerning symptoms of CM1 include those related to brainstem or upper cervical spinal cord compression. Medullary compression may adversely impact respiratory function and lead to sleep apnea, whereas similar brainstem or cervical spinal cord compression may cause sensorimotor deficits (hemiparesis, upper extremity paraparesis, quadriparesis), spasticity, or bladder dysfunction.[1–3,7,10,14] Additionally, lower cranial nerve deficits may present in up to 10% of pediatric patients with CM1, causing dysphagia, absent gag reflex, dysarthria, vocal cord dysfunction, or abnormal extraocular motility (eg, esotropia owing to cranial nerve VI paresis).[1,2,5,7,14] These symptoms occur with less frequency in the modern era likely owing to the advent of MRI offering earlier diagnosis, before neurologic disability occurs.[1,7] Medullary compression symptoms are also seen more commonly in children with complex CM1 that includes basilar invagination and/or instability with ventral compression of the cervicomedullary junction.[1,16] Up to 10% of patients with CM1 may also present with hydrocephalus owing to fourth ventricular outlet obstruction.[2,7]

CLINICAL PRESENTATION DURING THE NEONATAL PERIOD AND INFANCY (AGE 0 TO 3 YEARS)

Owing to limitations of communication, neonates or infants with symptomatic CM1 often present with generalized irritability.[2–5,7] Clinical signs that offer enhanced localization, as well as heightened concern, include opisthotonus, frequent neck extension/arching, and/or apneic episodes.[2–5,7] Additionally, crying spells with behavioral patterns suggesting head discomfort (reaching for the head or neck) may provide some amount of reliable localization.[5,7,14] Oropharyngeal dysfunction, owing to lower cranial nerve dysfunction, represents one of the most common presenting symptoms of children aged 0 to 2 years with CM1.[8,14] Medullary compression with lower cranial nerve dysfunction may manifest as[3,5,7,8,13,14,16]:

- Dysphagia, choking, or aspiration;
- Poor feeding, failure to thrive;
- Gastroesophageal reflux;
- Persistent cough;
- Snoring or episodic sleep apnea;
- Stridor; and
- Recurrent respiratory infections.

These more dramatic presentations reflect the underlying anatomic pathophysiology of cervicomedullary compression at the craniocervical junction, and are most typically observed in the setting of significant ventral compression owing to basilar invagination, retroflexion of the dens, and/or frank cervical instability.[16,17] Although occurring less frequently than in older children, clinical presentations with syringomyelia and/or scoliosis also are possible in the neonatal and infant populations.[3,8,14] In this and other age groups, there does not seem to exist a correlation between the extent of tonsillar herniation and the presence or absence of syringomyelia.[8]

CLINICAL PRESENTATION IN TODDLERS (AGE 3 TO 5 YEARS)

As patients develop improved ability to communicate and localize their pain, they may be able to verbalize more effectively complaints attributable to the presence of an underlying CM1. Toddlers with adequate verbal skills may report headache pain or discomfort in the upper neck. Occipital headaches represent a component of the clinical presentation of CM1 in up to 40% to 57% of patients during the toddler stages and early childhood.[2,3,8,14] Children aged 3 to 5 years with CM1 also may present frequently with syringomyelia and/or scoliosis (the latter present in 14%–38% of pediatric patients).[3,7,8,14,15] These patients may report back or shoulder pain, paresthesia, gait disturbance, and/or clumsiness. Alternatively, physical examination findings of cosmetic irregularity along the spine, subtle sensorimotor deficits, or hyperreflexia may reflect underlying scoliosis or syringomyelia. As with neonates and infants, symptoms or signs of medullary and lower cranial nerve dysfunction (sleep apnea, oropharyngeal dysphagia, dysarthria, absent gag reflex) may be present in toddlers with CM1.[7,8,12,14]

CLINICAL PRESENTATION DURING CHILDHOOD AND ADOLESCENCE (AGE 5 YEARS AND OLDER)

As they mature into the childhood and adolescent years, pediatric patients more frequently and reliably report the classic symptoms of CM1. Most commonly, patients note occipital headaches and/or neck pain, often induced by Valsalva-type maneuvers (straining for a bowel movement, laughing, coughing, sneezing, etc) and of short duration.[2] To warrant surgical consideration, these headaches should be severe enough to impact activities of daily living (ie, missing school) or quality of life.[5] As with younger patients (although less frequently), older children and adolescents with CM1 may experience oropharyngeal dysfunction.

Scoliosis, typically associated with syringomyelia (present in 19%–76% of CM1 patients), represents another important component of the clinical presentation in this group of patients.[1–3,8,9,14,15] Syringomyelia with scoliosis may lead to back or shoulder pain in children and adolescents.[2] Classic symptoms and physical examination signs suggesting syringomyelia include[5,7,10]:

- Upper extremity weakness, prominently affecting intrinsic muscles of the hand;
- Pain and temperature sensory loss (functions served by the spinal cord anterolateral spinothalamic tracts) in a 'cape-like' distribution;

- Preservation of light touch sensation and proprioception (functions served by the spinal cord dorsal columns); and
- Absence of superficial abdominal reflexes ipsilateral to the convexity of scoliosis.

As explained, the constellation of CM1, syringomyelia, and/or scoliosis may produce multiple physical examination findings that are easier to elicit or observe within children and adolescents (see **Table 1**). **Table 2** provides a summary of the more prominent clinical characteristics of CM1 and syringomyelia based on patient age.

Table 2
Prominent symptoms and signs of Chiari I malformation and syringomyelia in children, based on mechanism and age

Age Group	Cervicomedullary Compression, Impaired Cerebrospinal Fluid Flow Dynamics	Lower Cranial Nerve Dysfunction	Syringomyelia
Neonate and infant (age 0–3 y)	Generalized irritability Crying episodes, reaching for back of head or neck Respiratory dysfunction, sleep apnea, stridor Opisthotonus, neck arching Hydrocephalus	Oropharyngeal dysphagia, aspiration Poor feeding, failure to thrive Gastroesophageal reflux	Sensorimotor deficits (less frequent than older age groups)
Toddler (age 3–5 y)	Occipitocervical pain, prompted by Valsalva Respiratory dysfunction, sleep apnea, stridor Ataxia, gait dysfunction Hydrocephalus	Oropharyngeal dysphagia, aspiration Vocal cord dysfunction, hoarseness, dysarthria Absent/reduced gag reflex Extraocular motor deficits (eg, esotropia) Sensory loss in trigeminal distribution	Scoliosis Back or shoulder pain Upper extremity weakness, atrophy Lower extremity spasticity/hyperreflexia Dissociated sensory loss (pain/temperature) Absent superficial abdominal reflex
Childhood and adolescence (Age >5 y)	Occipitocervical pain, prompted by Valsalva Respiratory dysfunction, sleep apnea, stridor (less frequent than younger age groups) Dysesthetic pain in C2 dermatomal distribution Ataxia, gait dysfunction Hydrocephalus	Oropharyngeal dysfunction (less frequent than younger age groups) Vocal cord dysfunction, hoarseness, dysarthria Absent/reduced gag reflex Extraocular motor deficits (eg, esotropia) Sensory loss in trigeminal distribution	Scoliosis Back or shoulder pain Upper extremity weakness, impaired dexterity or fine motor control Lower extremity spasticity/hyperreflexia Dissociated sensory loss (pain/temperature) Absent superficial abdominal reflex

Table 3
Craniocervical and spinal osseous abnormalities associated with Chiari I malformation

Anatomic Location	Osseous Abnormality
Cranial vault	Decreased volume of posterior fossa
Craniocervical junction	Basilar invagination Platybasia Atlas assimilation
Cervical spine	Odontoid process retroversion/retro-flexion Klippel–Feil anomaly or variants
Vertebral column	Hemivertebra Butterfly vertebra

CLINICAL CONDITIONS ASSOCIATED WITH CHIARI I MALFORMATION

In addition to scoliosis, other, less common spinal or craniocervical osseous abnormalities may occur in the pediatric CM1 population (**Table 3**).[1–3,5–8,15–18] CM1 represents a common finding (up to 33%–38%) in patients with craniovertebral junction abnormalities like basilar invagination.[1] A variety of other clinical conditions and syndromes have been associated with CM1. The most common associated conditions include[2,3,5,7,8]:

- Hydrocephalus (8%–10%)[2,7];
- Neurofibromatosis type I (up to 5%)[2,7];
- Growth hormone deficiency (idiopathic; around 4%)[2,7];
- Sprengel deformity (abnormal elevation of the scapula); and
- Pierre Robin syndrome.

RARE PRESENTATIONS OF CHIARI I MALFORMATION IN CHILDREN

In addition to the common clinical presentations of CM1 described, more obscure presentations exist based on their acuity, rapid progression, or rarity of symptomatology. In unusual circumstances, pediatric patients with CM1 can present acutely in distress and require urgent operative intervention. Previously reported acute onset or rapidly progressive symptoms and signs include[2,19]:

- Dysphagia;
- Hemiparesis;
- Respiratory distress;
- Gait dysfunction; and
- Anisocoria.

These acutely presenting or rapidly progressive symptoms and signs reflect pathologic compression of the brainstem and/or spinal cord long

Table 4
Rare presentations of Chiari I malformation in children

Severity of Presentation	Clinical Finding
Mild	Nystagmus (typically downbeating) Chronic hiccoughs Chronic cough Cerebellar or cerebellovestibular dysfunction (eg, vertigo)
Moderate	Focal sensorimotor deficits (mononeuropathy; eg, plantar flexion weakness) Urinary incontinence Torticollis Trigeminal or glossopharyngeal neuralgia Sensorineural hearing loss
Severe	Syncopal episodes, drop attacks Acute spinal cord injury after trauma (eg, quadriplegia) Respiratory failure requiring mechanical ventilation Cardiorespiratory arrest, sudden death

tracts.[19] Although the specific symptoms may not represent rare findings (given their appearance as chronic symptoms in other CM1 patients), their rapid presentation or progression defy common patterns. Several rare presentations of CM1 have been reported in the literature and are summarized in **Table 4**.[2,3,5,7,8,10,12–15,19]

SUMMARY

CM1 and syringomyelia may be associated with a wide spectrum of symptoms and signs in children. Clinical presentations vary based on patient age and relative frequency, although some diagnoses of CM1 represent incidental radiographic findings in asymptomatic patients. Occipitocervical pain, propagated or intensified by Valsalva maneuvers (or generalized irritability in younger patients unable to communicate verbally), and syringomyelia with or without scoliosis represent the most common clinical presentations in the pediatric population. Cranial nerve or brainstem dysfunction also may be observed in younger patients, and is associated typically with more complex deformity that includes ventral compression secondary to basilar invagination, retroflexion of the dens, and/or craniocervical instability.

REFERENCES

1. Menezes AH. Craniovertebral junction abnormalities with hindbrain herniation and syringomyelia: regression of syringomyelia after removal of ventral craniovertebral junction compression. J Neurosurg 2012; 116(2):301–9.
2. Tubbs RS, Beckman J, Naftel RP, et al. Institutional experience with 500 cases of surgically treated pediatric Chiari malformation Type I. J Neurosurg Pediatr 2011;7(3):248–56.
3. Tubbs RS, McGirt MJ, Oakes WJ. Surgical experience in 130 pediatric patients with Chiari I malformations. J Neurosurg 2003;99(2):291–6.
4. Benglis D Jr, Covington D, Bhatia R, et al. Outcomes in pediatric patients with Chiari malformation Type I followed up without surgery. J Neurosurg Pediatr 2011;7(4):375–9.
5. Tubbs RS, Griessenauer CJ, Oakes WJ. Chiari malformations. In: Albright AL, Pollack IF, Adelson PD, editors. Principles and practice of pediatric neurosurgery. 3rd edition. New York: Thieme; 2015. p. 217–32.
6. Milhorat TH, Chou MW, Trinidad EM, et al. Chiari I malformation redefined: clinical and radiographic findings for 364 symptomatic patients. Neurosurgery 1999;44(5):1005–17.
7. Rozzelle CJ. Clinical presentation of pediatric Chiari I malformations. In: Tubbs RS, Oakes WJ, editors. The Chiari malformations. New York: Springer; 2013. p. 247–53.
8. Greenlee JD, Donovan KA, Hasan DM, et al. Chiari I malformation in the very young child: the spectrum of presentations and experience in 31 children under age 6 years. Pediatrics 2002;110(6):1212–9.
9. Muhonen MG, Menezes AH, Sawin PD, et al. Scoliosis in pediatric Chiari malformations without myelodysplasia. J Neurosurg 1992;77(1):69–77.
10. Laufer I, Engel M, Feldstein N, et al. Chiari malformation presenting as a focal motor deficit. Report of two cases. J Neurosurg Pediatr 2008;1(5):392–5.
11. Dahdaleh NS, Menezes AH. Incomplete lateral medullary syndrome in a patient with Chiari malformation Type I presenting with combined trigeminal and vagal nerve dysfunction. J Neurosurg Pediatr 2008;2(4):250–3.
12. Aitken LA, Lindan CE, Sidney S, et al. Chiari type I malformation in a pediatric population. Pediatr Neurol 2009;40(6):449–54.
13. Chambers KJ, Setlur J, Hartnick CJ. Chiari type I malformation: presenting as chronic cough in older children. Laryngoscope 2013;123(11):2888–91.
14. Albert GW, Menezes AH, Hansen DR, et al. Chiari malformation Type I in children younger than age 6 years: presentation and surgical outcome. J Neurosurg Pediatr 2010;5(6):554–61.
15. Greenlee J, Garell PC, Stence N, et al. Comprehensive approach to Chiari malformation in pediatric patients. Neurosurg Focus 1999;6(6):e4.
16. Bollo RJ, Riva-Cambrin J, Brockmeyer MM, et al. Complex Chiari malformations in children: an analysis of preoperative risk factors for occipitocervical fusion. J Neurosurg Pediatr 2012;10(2):134–41.
17. Goel A. Basilar invagination, Chiari malformation, syringomyelia: a review. Neurol India 2009;57(3):235–46.
18. Goel A, Desai K, Bhatjiwale M, et al. Basilar invagination and Chiari malformation associated with cerebellar atrophy: report of two treated cases. J Clin Neurosci 2002;9(2):194–6.
19. Wellons JC 3rd, Tubbs RS, Bui CJ, et al. Urgent surgical intervention in pediatric patients with Chiari malformation type I. Report of two cases. J Neurosurg 2007;107(1 Suppl):49–52.

Clinical Presentation and Alternative Diagnoses in the Adult Population

Ulrich Batzdorf, MD

KEYWORDS

- Adult • Tussive headaches • Alternative diagnoses • Syringomyelia

KEY POINTS

- Tussive headaches are reported in 80% to 100% of patients.
- When posterior fossa volume is reduced by basilar invagination, occipital cervical fusion may be required.
- Involution of the central canal in adulthood may explain why most adults do not present with syringomyelia.
- Symptoms can often present after minor trauma in the adult population.

SYMPTOMS IN THE ADULT CHIARI PATIENT

Adult patients with Chiari malformation, (Chiari 1 malformation), also termed cerebellar ectopia or hindbrain descent, classically present with strain-related headaches, which are reported to occur in 80% to 100 % of patients.[1] Typically these are brief, intense headaches, lasting a few seconds, located posteriorly at the base of the skull. They are generally reproducible with similar maneuvers, such as coughing (tussive headaches), straining, and lifting. Although they are characteristic, adults not uncommonly also have headaches of other etiologies, such as migraine headaches or neck pain radiating into the suboccipital area, which may coexist or overlap with more typical Chiari headaches. It is important to establish whether a Chiari patient has different types of headaches, if only to be clear that non-Chiari headaches will not be affected by surgery. This is particularly true in patients in whom tonsillar descent has been identified as an incidental finding on a study initially performed for other reasons, who do not present because of suspected Chiari-related symptoms.

Posterior headache and neck pain are also seen in patients with basilar invagination and with ligamentous instability at the craniocervical junction. The posterior fossa volume is characteristically reduced in patients with Chiari malformation. Volume also is reduced with basilar invagination, and true tonsillar descent may also be present in these patients. In some patients with basilar invagination, treatment may require craniocervical stabilization in addition to posterior fossa decompression.

Displacement and compression of the brainstem and stretching of lower cranial nerves can give rise to several other manifestations including nausea and vomiting and swallowing, as well as cough symptoms. Visual symptoms, including blurring of vision, double vision, and occasionally awareness of nystagmoid movements, are generally attributed to traction on cranial nerves III, IV, and VI, and their central connections. Tinnitus is often reported by Chiari patients. Patients also report balance problems and sleep disturbance. Findings on examination may include nystagmus, absence of venous pulsations on fundoscopic examination, and impaired truncal balance. The gag reflex may be absent. Facial pain may result from trigeminal nerve traction. Tongue fasciculations and hemiatrophy are sometimes encountered

Neurosurgery, Brain Research Institute, University of California, Los Angeles, Los Angeles, CA 90095, USA
E-mail address: UBatzdorf@mednet.ucla.edu

Neurosurg Clin N Am 26 (2015) 515–517
http://dx.doi.org/10.1016/j.nec.2015.07.001
1042-3680/15/$ – see front matter © 2015 Elsevier Inc. All rights reserved.

and are attributed to hypoglossal nerve traction. The anatomic basis of fatigue, memory impairment, and what patients sometimes refer to as brain fog is less clear. Findings related to syringomyelia may include upper extremity weakness and atrophy, sensory disturbances, and long-tract signs indicative of myelopathy. Autonomic symptoms, including postural hypotension, are sometimes seen in patients with Chiari malformation as well as in syringomyelia patients.

One assumes that the basic anatomic features, such as posterior fossa volume and size of the cerebellar hemispheres, have been established and stable by the time an individual has reached adult size. The question therefore arises frequently what it is that leads to the development of clinical symptoms in adult years, such as the headache described previously. One hypothesis is that years of normal activity, including coughing, lifting and straining, result in gradual downward displacement of the tonsils until there is interference with cerebrospinal fluid (CSF) flow at the level of the foramen magnum. The observation made in 1 study, that almost 25% of adult patients presenting with symptoms of tonsillar ectopia had a history of recent trauma,[1] is important in this connection, when one assumes that trauma can also result in critical downward displacement of marginally low cerebellar tonsils. Although symptom progression is gradual in most patients, occasionally symptoms related to Chiari malformation and even symptoms of syringomyelia may develop suddenly in relation to a severe coughing spell. Sudden death due to Chiari malformation is rare and is probably related to critical brainstem compression.[2,3] Without doubt there are also some individuals with Chiari malformation and even with associated syringomyelia, who remain minimally symptomatic their entire life.[4]

In a typical Chiari patient, the cerebellar tonsils are pointed and often peg-like at the C1 and sometimes the C 2 vertebral levels. Axial images at the foramen magnum will show obliteration of the subarachnoid space between tonsils and brainstem, and often show distortion of the brainstem by one or both tonsils. It must also be made clear that the designation of 5 mm tonsil projection below the foramen magnum as the critical measurement defining Chiari malformation is somewhat arbitrary.[5] Depending on some factors identified and others less clear, individuals may have normally rounded tonsils that project slightly more than 5 mm but cause no obstruction of CSF flow, while in other patients the configuration is such that reduced CSF flow can occur at the foramen magnum with less than 5 mm of tonsillar descent. It is also recognized that the precise

measurement of tonsil descent may vary with the degree of the patient's neck flexion or extension during the imaging study, which is difficult to reproduce exactly on sequential imaging studies. This is a consideration of importance when differences of a few millimeters of tonsil descent are reported on studies obtained at different times. It is also important to note that variations in posterior fossa architecture exist within the general concept of reduced posterior fossa volume in patients with Chiari malformation. Basilar invagination, with encroachment of the dens into the posterior fossa space, has already been mentioned. Other variations include a horizontally oriented occipital bone, low insertion of the tentorium cerebelli, and thickened skull bone.

Pulsatile motion of the brain, including the cerebellar tonsils, allows the tonsils to act as pistons, thereby forcing CSF into the spinal cord. This is postulated to be the mechanism of syringomyelia formation.[6] It has been suggested that persistence of the central canal of the cord, present at birth but not infrequently present in adults,[1,7] favors the development of syringomyelia. By contrast, involution of the central canal by the time critical descent of the tonsils occurs would explain why many adults have a Chiari malformation without syringomyelia.

Rarely syringomyelia is seen in patients without tonsillar descent who have a different abnormality impairing normal CSF outflow from the cranial cavity. Examples of such conditions are a retained rhombic roof over the fourth ventricle, or a postinflammatory or other obstructive membrane at the level of the foramen magnum. Such membranes may sometimes be identified by Constructive Interference with Steady State (CISS) imaging. This has sometimes been referred to as a Chiari zero malformation.[8]

ALTERNATIVE DIAGNOSES

Consideration of other diagnoses is particularly important in patients with atypical clinical presentation who have imaging features of tonsil descent interpreted as Chiari malformation, often based on a measurement. More persistent background headache, which, as any background headache, may be increased by coughing and straining, may be seen in patients with idiopathic intracranial hypertension (IIH), also known as pseudotumor cerebri. This diagnosis needs to be ruled out by appropriate ophthalmologic examination to determine whether there is papilledema, by imaging studies, and occasionally by direct intracranial pressure measurements. In such patients, posterior fossa decompression for tonsil descent, when IIH is overlooked, may be associated with a problematic outcome.

Tonsil descent can also be seen in patients with low CSF pressure in the spinal canal. Initially described in patients with lumbar CSF shunts,[9] this may also result from trauma, leakage of CSF related to prior spinal surgery, and occasionally from a dural opening of presumed congenital origin. Headache in such patients is often precipitated abruptly when the patient is upright and relieved in the recumbent position, and may be helped by increased fluid intake. Every effort must be made to identify the source of CSF leakage. Repair of such a leak usually results in ascent of the tonsils to a more normal position.

Other clinical entities may coexist with cerebellar tonsillar descent, and headaches may present in a similar manner. As such, they need to be considered in the evaluation of Chiari patients. Patients with a hereditary connective tissue disorder may exhibit excessive mobility between the skull and upper cervical spine,[10] with the result that the brainstem may be draped over the abnormally positioned odontoid process of the axis vertebra (C 2). Ehlers-Danlos syndrome is the best known of these conditions. Although the position of the odontoid contributes to the overall image of a smaller-than-normal posterior fossa, such patients often do not respond as well to posterior fossa decompression as do uncomplicated Chiari patients, and many require craniocervical fusion of some type to achieve symptom improvement.[11] Tethering of the spinal cord by a tight or fatty filum terminale may be associated with a finding of cerebellar tonsillar descent. When tonsil descent is seen with tethering related to spina bifida, even when a surgical closure has been performed, it is generally considered a Chiari 2 malformation.

SUMMARY

In a similar fashion to children, adult Chiari patients most commonly present with tussive headaches. They also present with lower cranial nerve dysfunction. The anatomic relationship of fatigue to Chiari 1 malformations is less than clear. The consideration of alternative diagnoses is important in adults and must be evaluated prior to considering surgical intervention.

REFERENCES

1. Milhorat TH, Chou MW, Trinidad EM, et al. Chiari I malformation redefined: clinical and radiographic findings for 364 symptomatic patients. Neurosurgery 1999;44:1005–17.
2. Friede RL, Roessman U. Chronic tonsillar herniation: an attempt at classifying chronic herniations at the foramen magnum. Acta Neuropathol 1976;34:219–35.
3. Williams B. Chronic herniation of the hindbrain. Ann R Coll Surg Engl 1981;63(1):9–17.
4. Meadows J, Kraut M, Guarnieri M, et al. Asymptomatic Chiari type 1 malformations identified on magnetic resonance imaging. J Neurosurg 2000;92:920–6.
5. Barkovich AJ, Wippold FJ, Sherman H, et al. Significance of cerebellar tonsillar position on MR. AJNR Am J Neuroradiol 1986;7:795–9.
6. Oldfield EH, Muraszko K, Shawker TH, et al. Pathophysiology of syringomyelia associated with Chiari I malformation of the cerebellar tonsils. J Neurosurg 1994;80:3–15.
7. Yasui K, Hashizume Y, Yoshida M, et al. Age-related morphologic changes of the central canal of the human spinal cord. Acta Neuropathol (Berl) 1999;97:253–9.
8. Iskandar BJ, Hedlund GL, Grabb PA, et al. The resolution of syringohydromyelia without hindbrain herniation after posterior fossa decompression. J Neurosurg 1998;80:212–6.
9. Hoffman HJ, Tucker WS. Cephalocranial disproportion. A complication of the treatment of hydrocephalus in children. Childs Brain 1976;2:167–76.
10. Milhorta TJ, Bolognese PA, Nishikawa M, et al. Syndrome of occipitoatlantoaxial hypermobility, cranial settling, and Chiari malformation type 1in patients with hereditary disorders of connective tissue. J Neurosurg Spine 2007;7:601–9.
11. Kim LJ, Rekate HL, Klopfenstein JD, et al. Treatment of basilar invagination associated with Chiari I malformation in the pediatric population: cervical reduction and posterior occipitocervical fusion. J Neurosurg 2004;101:189–95.

Advanced Imaging of Chiari 1 Malformations

Akbar Fakhri, MD[a], Manish N. Shah, MD[b,c], Manu S. Goyal, MD, MSc[a,*]

KEYWORDS

- Chiari malformation • Cerebrospinal fluid flow imaging • Cine fast image spin precession • MRI

KEY POINTS

- Advanced imaging in type I Chiari malformations currently includes cerebrospinal fluid (CSF) flow imaging, cerebellar tonsillar imaging at the foramen magnum, quantitative posterior fossa biometrics and volumetrics, and spinal cord diffusion tensor imaging.
- Patients with type I Chiari malformations may have increased CSF flow velocities, nonuniform axial plane CSF flow, different anterior and posterior foramen magnum CSF flow, and bidirectional CSF flow.
- Normalization of CSF flow parameters such as decreased maximal flow velocities may be correlated with better surgical outcome.
- Improvement in tonsillar pulsatility seen on cine fast image spin precession imaging is seen postoperatively.

 Videos of qualitative grading of differences between anterior and posterior flow accompany this article at http://www.neurosurgery.theclinics.com/

BACKGROUND

Type I Chiari malformation is a congenital deformity defined by caudal displacement of the cerebellar tonsils below the foramen magnum.[1–3] Routine brain and cervical spine MRI is sufficient to determine the position of the cerebellar tonsils. Additional anatomic changes may include small posterior fossa size with crowding at the foramen magnum. Standard T1- and T2-weighted sequences of the brain and spinal cord adequately evaluate for associated abnormalities including syrinx, hydrocephalus, and craniovertebral anomalies.[4–6] Patients with syringomyelia or marked cerebellar tonsillar descent may be symptomatic,[7] but these anatomic findings are neither sensitive nor specific.[8,9]

Advanced imaging in type I Chiari malformation aims to improve accurate assessment of the severity of type I Chiari malformation and its effects on cerebrospinal fluid (CSF) dynamics. The primary goals of advanced imaging in patients type I Chiari malformation are to

- Better predict whether the symptoms experienced by the patient are related to the type I Chiari malformation
- Determine the likelihood that posterior decompression will improve the patient's symptoms
- Improve understanding of the pathophysiology of type I Chiari malformation

Advanced imaging in type I Chiari malformation currently includes

- CSF flow imaging at the foramen magnum using cardiac-gated phase-contrast MRI

Disclosures: The authors have nothing to disclose.
[a] Mallinckrodt Institute of Radiology, Washington University School of Medicine, 1 Barnes Jewish Hospital Plaza, St Louis, MO 63110, USA; [b] Department of Pediatric Surgery, University of Texas, Health Science Center at Houston, 6431 Fannin Street, MSB 5.144, Houston, TX 77030, USA; [c] Department of Neurosurgery, University of Texas, Health Science Center at Houston, 6431 Fannin Street, MSB 5.144, Houston, TX 77030, USA
* Corresponding author.
E-mail address: goyalm@mir.wustl.edu

Neurosurg Clin N Am 26 (2015) 519–526
http://dx.doi.org/10.1016/j.nec.2015.06.012

- Cerebellar tonsillar motion at the foramen magnum using pulse-gated cine MRI
- Quantitative volumetrics of the posterior fossa and biometrics of the skull base
- Diffusion tensor imaging of the spinal cord

CSF dynamic studies at the foramen magnum are now routinely used to determine the severity of CSF flow disturbance. The degree of CSF flow disturbance has been shown to correlate with severity and development of clinical symptoms.[10] Furthermore, postoperative CSF flow imaging allows characterization of CSF flow normalization to assess surgical success. This article discusses CSF flow and cerebellar tonsillar motion imaging using MRI, acknowledging that newer techniques such as diffusion tensor imaging may have a role in the future.

RADIOLOGIC DIAGNOSIS

Tonsillar position in normal patients ranges from 8 mm above the foramen magnum to 5 mm below the foramen magnum.[5] Tonsillar displacement of 5 mm or more—with an age-dependent range of 5 mm in adults and 6 mm in children—is widely considered the criteria for type I Chiari malformation diagnosis. However, approximately 30% of patients with 5 to 10 mm of cerebellar tonsillar displacement will be asymptomatic, and some patients with 3 to 4 mm of cerebellar tonsillar displacement have been found to be symptomatic.[1]

Thus, the definition of type I Chiari malformation has varied across studies. However, the most widely used definitions include

- Less than 3 mm cerebellar tonsillar displacement below the foramen magnum is normal.
- Greater than 5 mm (in adults) displacement and greater than 6 mm (in children) is consistent with type I Chiari malformation.

Tonsillar displacement between 3 to 5 mm may be termed benign cerebellar ectopia or low-lying cerebellar tonsils and requires close correlation with other imaging findings and symptoms.[5] Furthermore, a peglike or pointed sergeant stripe appearance of displaced cerebellar tonsils on sagittal views with crowding at the foramen magnum helps to distinguish type I Chiari malformation from benign tonsillar ectopia. Measurements are typically taken from the lowest level of the foramen magnum to the lowest lying tonsil. Asymmetric tonsillar herniation is common, and the more displaced tonsil should be used for measurement.

Spine imaging is essential in initial evaluation because of the high percentage of associated syrinx formation. Syrinx formation is most common at the C4 through C6 levels,[11] but may occur anywhere along the spinal cord.[8] Syrinx formation may involve the length of the cord, resulting in a holocord syrinx, and there may be septations within the cavity. Patients with type I Chiari malformation may have hydrocephalus and multiple craniovertebral anomalies, including platybasia, occipitocervical assimilation, a short clivus, and scoliosis. The bulbar variant of type I Chiari malformation, or Chiari 1.5, involves brainstem herniation through the foramen magnum, perhaps caused by congential anomalous elevation of the foramen magnum. Of note, isolated cerebellar tonsillar displacement is not unique to type I Chiari malformation, and this can be seen in patients with intracranial hypotension as well as in patients with increased intracranial pressure.

ADVANCED IMAGING
Cerebrospinal Fluid Flow MRI

In addition to slow bulk flow, there is to-and-fro motion of CSF across the foramen magnum that is rhythmically synchronized with cardiac pulsation and respiratory variation.[12] When blood flow enters the brain during cardiac systole, the rigidity of the skull and noncompressibility of water requires that something exit the cranial cavity to maintain intracranial pressure (the Monro-Kellie Doctrine). The exit of CSF via the foramen magnum into the more compliant spinal cavity normally provides some of this relief, until diastole, when CSF is allowed to return back into the cranial cavity.

In type I Chiari malformation, restriction of CSF flow across the foramen magnum may limit the dampening of intracranial pressure changes during the cardiac cycle.[13–17] This could also impair CSF pressure dampening in other causes of transiently increased intracranial pressure, such as during coughing or Valsalva. Furthermore, restriction to CSF flow could generate higher velocities and turbulence, which could represent on etiologic factor for syrinx formation.[18,19] However, the understanding of the role of impaired CSF flow dynamics in manifestations of type I Chiari malformation continues to evolve.

The cardiac pulsation of CSF can be readily assessed using a combination of cardiac-gated MRI, which uses automated QRS wave detection with a cardiac monitor to average images temporally across multiple cardiac cycles, and phase-contrast MRI, which identifies phase shifts in the signals returning from moving protons that is proportional to their velocity.[14,20–22] Cardiac-gated phase-contrast MRI is frequently acquired with the following specifications:

- Electrocardiogram (EKG) gating of the cardiac cycle, though pulse gating can be used instead
- Acquisition in axial and sagittal planes centered at the foramen magnum
- Setting of the initial maximum anticipated CSF flow velocity (VENC) to 5 to 10 cm/s
- Repeat study with higher VENC when it causes aliasing or lower VENC if CSF flow cannot be adequately visualized

Conventionally, velocity in the superior-to-inferior direction demonstrates bright signal, and velocity in the inferior-to-superior direction demonstrates dark signal. A region of interest can be placed at or directly below the foramen magnum anteriorly and posteriorly to quantitate CSF velocity.

The volume of CSF moving through the foramen magnum depends primarily on changes in cerebral blood volume. However, the velocity of fluid moving through the foramen magnum depends on the dimensions and crowding of the foramen magnum.[12] Hence, processes that restrict the flow within the foramen magnum will likely increase the velocity of flow rather than the volume of flow. In normal patients, the CSF flow is usually equivalent anterior and posterior to the cord throughout the cardiac cycle. Moreover, the flow in normal patients is uniform in either direction without aliasing in any region of interest. One study of systolic and diastolic velocities in normal patients showed an average peak systolic velocity of 2.4 cm/s and average peak diastolic velocity of 2.8 cm/s.[23]

Patients with type I Chiari malformation may demonstrate several abnormalities in CSF flow:

- Increased velocities: 1 study of systolic and diastolic velocities in patients with type I Chiari malformation demonstrated peak systolic velocity of 3.1 cm/s and peak diastolic velocity of 4.0 cm/s[23]
- Nonuniformity: flow may be nonuniform, particularly in the axial plane, secondary to

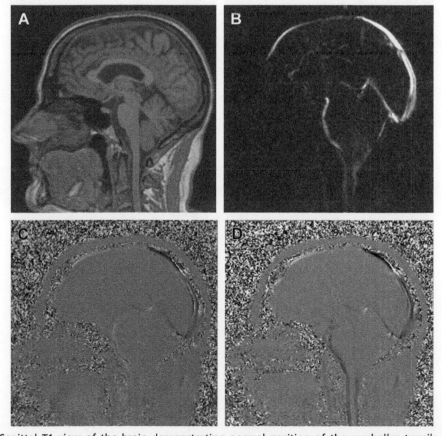

Fig. 1. (*A*) Sagittal T1 view of the brain demonstrating normal position of the cerebellar tonsils. (*B*) Sagittal second phase contrast image with a VENC of 10 showing normal flow at the foramen magnum anteriorly and posteriorly. (*C, D*) Midsagittal images from cine phase contrast study with a VENC of 10 showing bidirectional flow at the foramen magnum anteriorly and posteriorly.

mechanical obstruction throughout the cardiac cycle

- Differences between anterior and posterior flow: as the degree of flow restriction increases, flow is typically first impaired posteriorly and then increasingly anterior to the craniocervical junction. Qualitative grading of this finding has been shown to correlate with symptomatic type I Chiari malformation and is demonstrated in **Figs. 1–4** and Videos 1–6.
- Bidirectional flow: in type I Chiari malformation, CSF flow may occur caudally and cranially simultaneously, often visualized as focal aliasing despite a high VENC.

Cine MRI of Tonsillar Motion

In normal patients, there is slight caudal movement of the cerebellar tonsils followed by the medulla and spinal cord. Additionally, there is anteroposterior movement of the tonsils, medulla, and spinal cord. In patients with type I Chiari malformation, the changes in velocity are also accompanied by abnormal movements of the brainstem and upper spinal cord.

Cine MRI using a rapid image acquisition sequence, true fast image spin precession (true-FISP), coupled with pulse or cardiac gating, can identify pulsatile motion of brain structures during the cardiac cycle. This technique identifies increased pulsatile craniocaudal displacement of the cerebellar tonsils and upper cord in patients with type I Chiari malformation, which may correlate with type I Chiari malformation-specific symptoms.[15,24] Impaired passive recoil secondary to herniated tonsils can further contribute to CSF flow abnormality. In addition, abnormal posterior movement of the medulla may be seen while the tonsils move caudally and anteriorly. Upward motion is rarely seen. The downward displacement starts early in the cardiac cycle. One study demonstrated a greater tonsillar motion in patients with cough-associated headaches.[25] The motion of

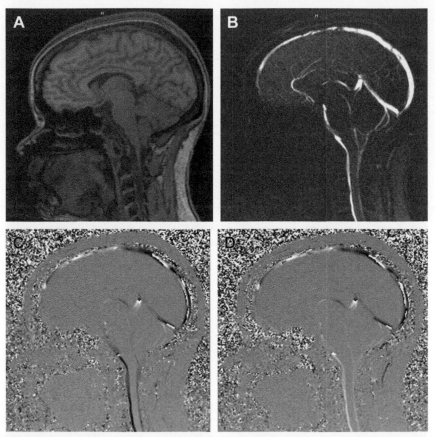

Fig. 2. (A) Sagittal T1 view of the brain showing type I Chiari malformation with peg-like shape of cerebellar tonsils and approximately 9 mm cerebellar tonsillar ectopia. (B) Sagittal second phase contrast image with a VENC of 10 showing normal flow with increased velocity at the foramen magnum anteriorly and posteriorly. (C, D) Midsagittal images from cine phase contrast study with a VENC of 10 showing normal bidirectional flow with increased velocity at the foramen magnum anteriorly and posteriorly.

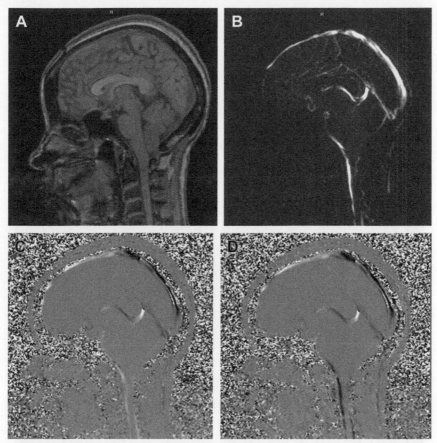

Fig. 3. (*A*) Sagittal T1 image of the brain demonstrating type I Chiari malformation with 7 mm cerebellar tonsillar ectopia. (*B*) Sagittal second phase contrast image of the brain with a VENC of 10 demonstrating normal flow anterior to the foramen magnum but markedly diminished flow posterior to foramen magnum. (*C, D*) Midsagittal images from cine phase contrast study with a VENC of 10 showing bidirectional flow anterior to the foramen magnum but no flow posterior to the foramen magnum.

the cerebellar tonsils and brainstem may also contribute to syrinx formation. In patients with type I Chiari malformation, the upper part of the cord is compressed, and syringes usually extend below the level of compression.

Diffusion Tensor Imaging

In addition to assessing flow and pulsatility with advanced MRI, diffusion tensor imaging (DTI) detects subtle white matter integrity changes before potential visualization on standard structural MRI. Quantitatively measuring the directional diffusion of free water with DTI for white matter tracts obtains fractional anisotropy and mean diffusivity. These fractional anisotrophy and mean diffusivity measures allow for quantitative white matter comparison early in the course of neurologic diseases such as depression[26] and hydrocephalus.[27] With regard to cervical syringomyelia, Hatem and colleagues[28] examined 28 patients and found lower

fractional anisotrophy values with somatosensory symptoms. DTI is another promising quantitative imaging tool to investigate the relationship of symptomatology to type I Chiari malformation with syringomyelia.

Postsurgical Outcome

Some patients may have no relief of clinical symptoms after decompressive surgery. CSF flow abnormalities may better select patients most likely to get a favorable response to surgery.[7,10] Normal preoperative CSF flow at the foramen magnum has been shown to be a risk factor for postdecompression failure, with 1 study showing patients with normal CSF flow parameters to be 4.8 times more likely to experience treatment failure.[10]

Symptomatic patients undergoing decompressive surgery involving suboccipital craniectomy, C1 laminectomy, and duroplasty may have normalization of CSF flow parameters seen on

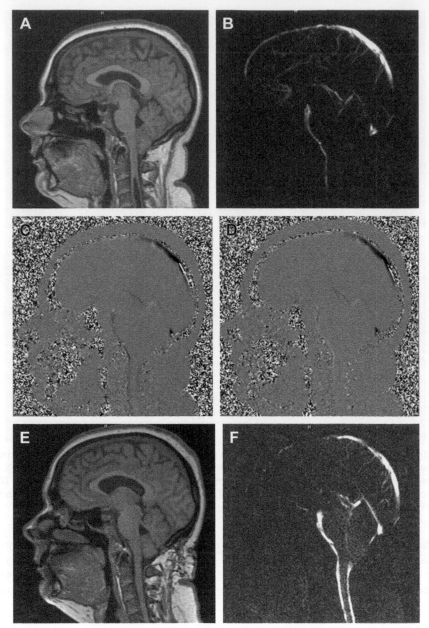

Fig. 4. (*A*) Sagittal T1 image in a patient with type I Chiari malformation with approximately 10 mm of cerebellar tonsillar ectopia. Also partially visualized is a syrinx starting at the C3 level and extending inferiorly. (*B–D*) Sagittal phase contrast imaging with a VENC of 10 demonstrating normal bidirectional flow anterior to the foramen magnum and absent flow posterior to the foramen magnum. (*E*) Sagittal T1 image of the same patient 2 years after posterior decompression surgery with removal of the posterior arch of C1. Interval resolution of previously seen syrinx at the C3 level. (*F–H*) Postoperative midsagittal phase contrast imaging with a VENC of 10 showing markedly improved bidirectional CSF flow posterior to the foramen magnum.

phase contrast imaging.[29] Normalization of CSF flow parameters has been correlated with improved clinical symptoms. Stabilization or reduction in syrinx size is also seen in the majority of patients after decompression. Overall, patients with worse preoperative CSF flow abnormalities show a better clinical response to decompressive surgery.[10]

Additionally, cardiac-gated true-FISP MRI holds promise for perioperative evaluation of type I Chiari malformation. This technique demonstrated moderate agreement among 3 reviewers for qualitative tonsillar pulsatility improvement with definite quantitative improvement, but, like all MRI paradigms, it is affected by postoperative artifacts.[11]

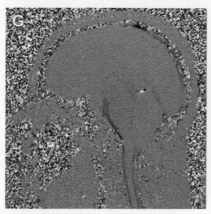
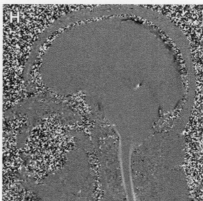

Fig. 4. (*continued*)

SUMMARY

Advanced imaging of type I Chiari malformation continues to evolve. Currently, CSF flow imaging using cardiac-gated phase-contrast MRI is now routinely performed to evaluate for CSF flow restriction at the foramen magnum. Abnormalities in pulsatile CSF flow across the foramen magnum help identify symptomatic patients. It may also help predict which patients will respond to posterior decompression, although further research is needed to determine this. Other techniques, such as cardiac-gated true-FISP MRI of tonsillar and brainstem motion and DTI, are increasingly used and may demonstrate utility in the management of type I Chiari malformation.

SUPPLEMENTARY DATA

Supplementary data related to this article can be found online at http://dx.doi.org/10.1016/j.nec. 2015.06.012.

REFERENCES

1. Barkovich A, Wippold FJ, Sherman JL, et al. Significance of cerebellar tonsillar position on MR. AJNR Am J Neuroradiol 1986;7(5):795–9.

2. Ishikawa M, Kikuchi H, Fujisawa I, et al. Tonsillar herniation on magnetic resonance imaging. Neurosurgery 1988;22(1):77–81.

3. Spinos E, Laster DW, Moody DM, et al. MR evaluation of Chiari I malformations at 0.15 T. AJNR Am J Neuroradiol 1985;6(2):203–8.

4. Caldarelli M, Di Rocco C. Diagnosis of Chiari I malformation and related syringomyelia: radiological and neurophysiological studies. Childs Nerv Syst 2004;20(5):332–5.

5. Chiapparini L, Saletti V, Solero CL, et al. Neuroradiological diagnosis of Chiari malformations. Neurol Sci 2011;32(3):283–6.

6. Elster AD, Chen M. Chiari I malformations: clinical and radiologic reappraisal. Radiology 1992;183(2): 347–53.

7. Hekman KE, Aliaga L, Straus D, et al. Positive and negative predictors for good outcome after decompressive surgery for Chiari malformation type 1 as scored on the Chicago Chiari Outcome Scale. Neurol Res 2012;34(7):694–700.

8. Godzik J, Kelly MP, Radmanesh A, et al. Relationship of syrinx size and tonsillar descent to spinal deformity in Chiari malformation Type I with associated syringomyelia. J Neurosurg Pediatr 2014;13(4):368–74.

9. Yarbrough CK, Greenberg JK, Smyth MD, et al. External validation of the Chicago Chiari Outcome Scale. J Neurosurg Pediatr 2014;13(6):679–84.

10. McGirt MJ, Nimjee SM, Fuchs HE, et al. Relationship of cine phase-contrast MRI to outcome after decompressionfor Chiari I malformation. Neurosurgery 2006;59(1):140–6.

11. Radmanesh A, Greenberg JK, Chatterjee A, et al. Tonsillar pulsatility before and after surgical decompression for children with Chiari malformation type 1: an application for true fast imaging with steady state precession. Neuroradiology 2015;57(4):387–93.

12. Haughton V, Mardal K-A. Spinal fluid biomechanics and imaging: an update for neuroradiologists. AJNR Am J Neuroradiol 2014;35(10):1864–9.

13. Bhadelia RA, Bogdan AR, Wolpert SM, et al. Cerebrospinal fluid flow waveforms: analysis in patients with Chiari I malformation by means of gated phase-contrast MR imaging velocity measurements. Radiology 1995;196(1):195–202.

14. Wolpert SM, Bhadelia RA, Bogdan AR, et al. Chiari I malformations: assessment with phase-contrast velocity MR. AJNR Am J Neuroradiol 1994;15(7):1299–308.

15. Ventureyra EC, Aziz HA, Vassilyadi M. The role of cine flow MRI in children with Chiari I malformation. Childs Nerv Syst 2003;19(2):109–13.

16. Quigley MF, Iskandar B, Quigley ME, et al. Cerebrospinal fluid flow in foramen magnum: temporal and

spatial patterns at MR imaging in volunteers and in patients with Chiari I malformation 1. Radiology 2004;232(1):229–36.

17. Shah S, Haughton V, del Río AM. CSF flow through the upper cervical spinal canal in Chiari I malformation. AJNR Am J Neuroradiol 2011;32(6):1149–53.

18. Brugières P, Idy-Peretti I, Iffenecker C, et al. CSF flow measurement in syringomyelia. AJNR Am J Neuroradiol 2000;21(10):1785–92.

19. Pinna G, Alessandrini F, Alfieri A, et al. Cerebrospinal fluid flow dynamics study in Chiari I malformation: implications for syrinx formation. Neurosurg Focus 2000;8(3):1–8.

20. Battal B, Kocaoglu M, Bulakbasi N, et al. Cerebrospinal fluid flow imaging by using phase-contrast MR technique. Turk Neurosurg 2014;84(1004): 758–65.

21. Hofmann E, Warmuth-Metz M, Bendszus M, et al. Phase-contrast MR imaging of the cervical CSF and spinal cord: volumetric motion analysis in patients with Chiari I malformation. AJNR Am J Neuroradiol 2000;21(1):151–8.

22. Mauer UM, Gottschalk A, Mueller C, et al. Standard and cardiac-gated phase-contrast magnetic resonance imaging in the clinical course of patients with Chiari malformation Type I. Neurosurg Focus 2011;31(3):E5.

23. Haughton VM, Korosec FR, Medow JE, et al. Peak systolic and diastolic CSF velocity in the foramen magnum in adult patients with Chiari I malformations and in normal control participants. Am J Neuroradiol 2003;24(2):169–76.

24. Pujol J, Roig C, Capdevila A, et al. Motion of the cerebellar tonsils in Chiari type I malformation studied by cine phase-contrast MRI. Neurology 1995; 45(9):1746–53.

25. Bhadelia R, Frederick E, Patz S, et al. Cough-associated headache in patients with Chiari I malformation: CSF flow analysis by means of cine phase-contrast MR imaging. AJNR Am J Neuroradiol 2011;32(4): 739–42.

26. Shimony JS, Sheline YI, D'Angelo G, et al. Diffuse microstructural abnormalities of normal-appearing white matter in late life depression: a diffusion tensor imaging study. Biol Psychiatry 2009;66(3):245–52.

27. Williams VJ, Juranek J, Stuebing KK, et al. Postshunt lateral ventricular volume, white matter integrity, and intellectual outcomes in spina bifida and hydrocephalus. J Neurosurg Pediatr 2015;15(4):410–9.

28. Hatem SM, Attal N, Ducreux D, et al. Assessment of spinal somatosensory systems with diffusion tensor imaging in syringomyelia. J Neurol Neurosurg Psychiatry 2009;80(12):1350–6.

29. Lee A, Yarbrough CK, Greenberg JK, et al. Comparison of posterior fossa decompression with or without duraplasty in children with Type I Chiari malformation. Childs Nerv Syst 2014;30(8):1419–24.

Surgical Treatment of Chiari I Malformation

Brandon G. Rocque, MD, MS, Walter Jerry Oakes, MD*

KEYWORDS

- Chiari I malformation • Posterior fossa decompression • Duraplasty • Surgical technique

KEY POINTS

- Anatomic Chiari I malformation is common, so selection of patients likely to benefit from posterior fossa decompression is crucial.
- Soft tissue dissection need not extend more lateral than the level of the lateral edge of the foramen magnum, thus lowering the risk of vertebral artery injury.
- Dural opening should proceed from caudal to rostral to allow greatest control of potential venous lakes in the occipital dura.
- Bone-only decompression has a higher risk of requiring repeat operation for lack of improvement, whereas decompression with duraplasty has a higher rate of cerebrospinal fluid (CSF) complications. No definitive evidence favors either technique.
- Assuring adequate CSF outflow from the fourth ventricle should be the primary goal, especially in redo Chiari decompression.

Videos of the Soft tissue dissection and bone removal for standard Chiari decompression; Dural opening and 4th ventricle exploration; and Redo Chiari decompression showing scarring of the 4th ventricle outlet accompany this article at http://www.neurosurgery.theclinics.com/

INTRODUCTION: NATURE OF THE PROBLEM

The Chiari I malformation is characterized by low position of the tonsils of the cerebellum. The definition of Chiari I is typically expressed by a measurement of the distance that the most inferior tip of the cerebellar tonsil lies below the foramen magnum. However, the prevalence of Chiari I malformation, based on this anatomic definition, is potentially as high as 1% of the general population.[1] However, only a small proportion of these Chiari I malformations are symptomatic or cause secondary pathologic phenomena like syringomyelia. The only accepted treatment for patients with symptomatic Chiari I malformation is surgical decompression of the hindbrain.

Although the typical symptoms of Chiari I malformation and syringomyelia, as well as the indications for undertaking surgical treatment, are discussed elsewhere in this issue, we briefly cover them here. The presence of a syrinx seems to be reasonable justification for operation.[2] Although some patients have been shown to have spontaneous syrinx resolution, the decision for surgery rests with the likelihood that a fixed neurologic deficit as a consequence of the syrinx is more probable than spontaneous syrinx resolution.[3]

In the absence of syringomyelia, an indication for operative treatment of the Chiari I malformation is often the presence of headache. Headaches that most reliably improve with Chiari I decompression are occipital or high cervical, are reproducibly brought on with Valsalva maneuver, and are of short duration. Relief of headaches that do not meet all of these criteria is less likely.

Department of Neurosurgery, University of Alabama at Birmingham, 1600 Seventh Avenue South, Lowder 400, Birmingham, AL 35233, USA
* Corresponding author.
E-mail address: jerry.oakes@childrensal.org

Neurosurg Clin N Am 26 (2015) 527–531
http://dx.doi.org/10.1016/j.nec.2015.06.010
1042-3680/15/$ – see front matter © 2015 Elsevier Inc. All rights reserved.

The purpose of this article is not to discuss indications for surgical treatment of Chiari I malformation. Rather, herein we describe the surgical technique and nuance for the operative treatment of the Chiari I malformation, including preoperative planning, patient positioning, surgical approach, the detailed surgical procedure, postoperative care, and recovery. We include a brief discussion of controversies surrounding opening of the dura and manipulation of the cerebellar tonsils, but the bulk of this text is a description of the surgical technique preferred at the authors' institution.

SURGICAL TECHNIQUE
Preoperative Planning

Before surgery, a detailed history and physical examination, routine preoperative laboratory evaluation, and pre-anesthetic risk profiling are performed. It is important that before surgery, patients and families understand the goals of surgical therapy. In the patient with syringomyelia, the goal is most often to prevent future neurologic deficit and to affect a decrease in the size of the syrinx. In the patient with headaches, the goal of therapy is to reduce the frequency and severity of the headaches that are attributable to the Chiari, as described previously. When the patient and family accept the risks and potential benefits of surgery, Chiari I decompression can proceed.

Preparation and Patient Positioning

The patient is positioned prone on a standard operating table with the head flexed (**Fig. 1**). Gel rolls or appropriate padding is used to support the chest and hips, leaving the abdomen free to facilitate ventilation. The head is secured using pin fixation. Pin fixation is an option in infants, particularly if a combination face support/pin fixation device is available. This type of device allows the weight of the infant's head to be supported by the forehead support, while the pins maintain the flexed position required for optimal surgical exposure.

Surgical Procedure

Step 1: soft tissue dissection
After standard surgical preparation and draping, a midline incision is made extending from just below the inion to the spinous process of the C2 vertebra. Most surgeons prefer to continue the dissection in the midline avascular plane down to the level of the occipital bone.

We generally perform exposure of the occipital bone first, including defining the borders of the foramen magnum. We then dissect the posterior arch of the C1 vertebra in a subperiosteal fashion. The goal of surgery is decompression of the hindbrain at the foramen magnum, and as such, lateral dissection is not necessary beyond that required to provide sufficient exposure of the lateral edges of the foramen magnum (approximately 1.5 cm off of midline bilaterally). Therefore, there is no need for significant lateral dissection of the occiput or C1 (**Fig. 2**). Refraining from excessive lateral dissection will help prevent injury to the vertebral artery, particularly in the presence of bony anomalies of the skull base and C1, when the course of the vertebral artery around C1 is less predictable.[4] It is rarely necessary to expose the bony elements

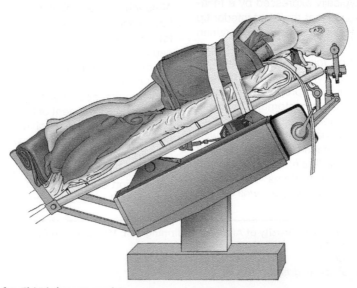

Fig. 1. Positioning for Chiari decompression.

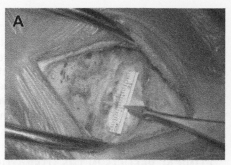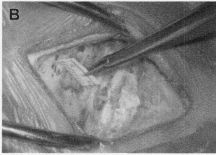

Fig. 2. Extent of exposure needed for Chiari decompression. (*A*) Ruler shows 2.5 cm of the posterior arch of C1 exposed; (*B*) 2.5 cm of occipital bone superior to foramen magnum is exposed.

of C2. Release of the muscle attachments from the inferior surface of the C2 spinous process and lamina may increase the risk of postoperative kyphotic deformity.[5]

Step 2: bony decompression

Bony opening is then performed. This can be accomplished with a high-speed drill or craniotome and rongeurs. When making the initial skull perforations with the drill, it is advisable to place bur holes off of midline, as there often exists a midline keel of variable depth. If a bur hole is placed on either side of this keel, then dissection can proceed toward the midline, and resection of the keel can be performed in a controlled fashion. The width of the bony opening should be the same as the width of the foramen magnum, usually 22 to 25 mm. This should be readily apparent as the point where the dura at the foramen magnum begins to curve into a vertical orientation. Restriction of the size of the craniectomy to approximately 22 to 25 mm superior to the foramen magnum should lower the risk of cerebellar slump, a condition that may lead to insidious return of Chiari symptoms.[6]

The posterior arch of C1 is then removed with either a high-speed drill or rongeur. If a rongeur is used, care must be taken to take clean bites without twisting, as the anterior ligamentous structures can be damaged by aggressive manipulation of C1 (Video 1).

Step 3: dural opening

Opening of the dura is typically performed in a caudal to rostral fashion. In the spine, caudal to the level of the foramen magnum, the dura is usually a single layer, whereas cranial dura has 2 layers. Dural sinuses lie between these 2 layers. An occipital sinus or significant venous lakes can exist between the layers of the dura over the posterior fossa, especially in infants. Opening first at the level of the C1 laminectomy places the initial opening at a spot where there are typically no venous structures. Dural opening can then

proceed rostrally, maintaining hemostasis by applying bipolar electrocautery before opening or by applying Weck clips or suture on each side as the dura is opened (**Fig. 3**). A vertical dural opening extending the length of the incision is usually sufficient. If there still appears to be compression, then a horizontal ramus of the incision can be made at the point of maximum constriction. Dura is retracted with the use of sutures. Arachnoid opening can then be performed sharply. Using Weck clips to affix the arachnoid to the cut dural edge at the time of opening will then facilitate closure of the arachnoid along with the dura. This maneuver helps to prevent accumulation of cerebrospinal fluid (CSF) in the extra-arachnoidal space that may lead to fourth ventricle outlet obstruction and hydrocephalus.[7] Care is taken to avoid contamination of the subarachnoid space with blood, thus limiting the formation of postoperative arachnoid adhesions and gliosis (Video 2).

Step 4: ensuring adequacy of fourth ventricle outlet

In 6% to 10% of cases, an arachnoidal veil can be found obstructing the outlet of the fourth

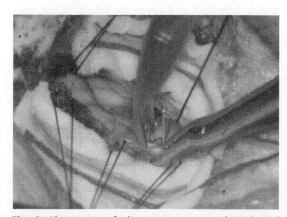

Fig. 3. Placement of clip to appose arachnoid and dura, preventing accumulation of CSF in the extra-arachnoid, subdural space.

ventricle.[8] After opening of the dura and arachnoid, the tonsils can be gently separated to inspect the fourth ventricle outlet; the goal being to visualize the floor of the fourth ventricle. When a veil of arachnoid is encountered, it can be carefully penetrated with fine forceps.

In highly symptomatic patients, those with very large syrinx, or those whose cerebellar tonsils extend significantly below the level of the dural opening, reduction of the cerebellar tonsils is an option to ensure adequate CSF outflow from the fourth ventricle. The senior author's preferred method is to incise the tonsils laterally/dorsally and to coagulate and aspirate the tonsils until they are reduced. This method avoids coagulation or manipulation of the medial pia of the tonsils, thus reducing the risk of postoperative scarring of the ventricular outlet.

Another alternative to ensure patency of the fourth ventricular outlet is the placement of a stent. A silastic tube, similar to that used for ventriculo-peritoneal shunting, can be placed with one end in the fourth ventricle and the other in the ventral cervical subarachnoid space (Video 3). This ensures a conduit for the flow of CSF out of the ventricular system. This method can be useful particularly for repeat Chiari decompression in a patient whose syrinx has recurred or worsened, possibly due to scarring at the fourth ventricular outlet.[9,10] If a stent is placed, it is important to secure the stent, for example by suturing it to the pia of the tonsil, lest it become dislodged.

Step 5: closure of the dura

Most investigators recommend closure of the dura, and there are a plethora of available materials.[11] Use of autologous tissue requires steps to harvest but avoids the possibility of reaction to the graft material. Use of a commercial dural substitute carries the theoretic risk of an immune reaction or infection, but saves the time of autologous tissue harvest. The authors' preference is autologous pericranium. This can be harvested via an extension of the surgical incision, although we prefer a second incision placed a few centimeters superior to the primary incision. Regardless of the material used, the goal is a watertight closure to prevent the formation of a pseudomeningocele, the most common complication after Chiari decompression surgery.[12] The remainder of the wound is closed in the standard fashion.

Postoperative Care

The patient is monitored in an intensive care or intermediate care setting overnight and is generally ready for discharge in 2 to 3 days. Scheduled nonnarcotic pain medication, ibuprofen and acetaminophen in alternating doses, has been shown to provide better postoperative analgesia with shorter length of stay than as-needed dosing of narcotics.[13] Rehabilitation is tailored to the needs of the patient, with most patients not requiring focused rehabilitation. Those patients with neurologic deficits secondary to syringomyelia are referred to physical or occupational therapy as needed.

CLINICAL RESULTS IN THE LITERATURE

Results of Chiari decompression are generally favorable. Improvement of symptoms is reported in 60% to 100% of patients in published series, and resolution of syringomyelia is reported to have a similar rate of success.[8,14–16] Debate is ongoing regarding the risks and benefits of posterior fossa decompression (PFD) alone versus posterior fossa decompression with duraplasty (PFDD). However, 2 meta-analyses along with many single-institution studies show no convincing evidence that one method is superior over the other.[14,15] In the meta-analysis performed by Durham and Fjeld-Olenec,[14] PFD had a significantly higher rate of reoperation (12.6% vs 2.1%) and lower rate of CSF-related complications (1.8% vs 18.5%) than PFDD. Based on the observation that 6% to 10% of patients will have an intradural finding that precludes free flow of CSF out of the fourth ventricle, it is the authors' opinion that intradural exploration is warranted as long as the surgeon's rate of CSF complication from this approach is less than approximately 5%.[17]

SUMMARY

Surgical decompression of the posterior fossa for treatment of Chiari I malformation is an operation with a high rate of success in properly selected patients. In this article, we presented techniques that we believe lead to the highest likelihood of good outcome (ie, resolution of typical Chiari-related symptoms and resolution of syringomyelia), as well as avoidance of complications.

SUPPLEMENTARY DATA

Supplementary data related to this article can be found online at http://dx.doi.org/10.1016/j.nec.2015.06.010.

REFERENCES

1. Vernooij MW, Ikram MA, Tanghe HL, et al. Incidental findings on brain MRI in the general population. N Engl J Med 2007;357:1821–8.

2. Rocque BG, George TM, Kestle J, et al. Treatment practices for Chiari malformation type I with syringomyelia: results of a survey of the American Society of Pediatric Neurosurgeons. J Neurosurg Pediatr 2011; 8:430–7.

3. Doughty KE, Tubbs RS, Webb D, et al. Delayed resolution of Chiari I-associated hydromyelia after posterior fossa decompression: case report and review of the literature. Neurosurgery 2004;55:711.

4. Tubbs RS, Smyth MD, Wellons JC 3rd, et al. Distances from the atlantal segment of the vertebral artery to the midline in children. Pediatr Neurosurg 2003;39(6):330–4.

5. McLaughlin MR, Wahlig JB, Pollack IF. Incidence of postlaminectomy kyphosis after Chiari decompression. Spine 1997;22:613–7.

6. Holly LT, Batzdorf U. Management of cerebellar ptosis following craniovertebral decompression for Chiari I malformation. J Neurosurg 2001;94:21–6.

7. Elton S, Tubbs RS, Wellons JC, et al. Acute hydrocephalus following a Chiari I decompression. Pediatr Neurosurg 2002;36:101–4.

8. Tubbs RS, Beckman J, Naftel RP, et al. Institutional experience with 500 cases of surgically treated pediatric Chiari malformation Type I. J Neurosurg Pediatr 2011;7:248–56.

9. Sacco D, Scott RM. Reoperation for Chiari malformations. Pediatr Neurosurg 2003;39:171–8.

10. Tubbs RS, Webb DB, Oakes WJ. Persistent syringomyelia following pediatric Chiari I decompression: radiological and surgical findings. J Neurosurg 2004;100:460–4.

11. Sonntag VH, Abla A, Link T, et al. Comparison of dural grafts in Chiari decompression surgery: review of the literature. J Craniovertebr Junction Spine 2010;1:29.

12. Parker SR, Harris P, Cummings TJ, et al. Complications following decompression of Chiari malformation Type I in children: dural graft or sealant? J Neurosurg Pediatr 2011;8:177–83.

13. Smyth MD, Banks JT, Tubbs RS, et al. Efficacy of scheduled nonnarcotic analgesic medications in children after suboccipital craniectomy. J Neurosurg 2004;100:183–6.

14. Durham SR, Fjeld-Olenec K. Comparison of posterior fossa decompression with and without duraplasty for the surgical treatment of Chiari malformation Type I in pediatric patients: a meta-analysis. J Neurosurg Pediatr 2008;2:42–9.

15. Hankinson T, Tubbs RS, Wellons JC. Duraplasty or not? An evidence-based review of the pediatric Chiari I malformation. Childs Nerv Syst 2010;27:35–40.

16. Krieger MD, McComb JG, Levy ML. Toward a simpler surgical management of Chiari I malformation in a pediatric population. Pediatr Neurosurg 1999;30:113–21.

17. Tubbs RS, Smyth MD, Wellons JC III. Arachnoid veils and the Chiari I malformation. J Neurosurg 2004;100:465–7.

Clinical Outcome Measures in Chiari I Malformation

Chester K. Yarbrough, MD, MPHS[a],*,
Jacob K. Greenberg, MD, MSCI[a], Tae Sung Park, MD[a,b]

KEYWORDS

- Chiari malformation type 1 • Outcome methods • Treatment outcome • Clinical research
- Outcome instruments • Quality of life

KEY POINTS

- Several commonly used general outcome measures have been used to evaluate treatment outcomes for patients with Chiari malformation type 1 (CM-I).
- Of the general quality of life and disability scales, the Neck Disability Index (NDI) and the Short Form (SF)-12 have been shown to have the most validity in patients with CM-I.
- Of the disease-specific outcome instruments, scales designed for use in patients with cervical spine problems, such as the modified Japanese Orthopaedic Association (JOA) score, have been used in the CM-I population. Although several of these scales adequately assess neurologic function related to CM-I, none assess all aspects of CM-I symptoms.
- Chiari-specific scales, such as the Chicago Chiari Outcome Scale (CCOS) and the Chiari Symptom Profile, assess the aspects of CM-I disease and treatment outcomes more completely than previous instruments.

INTRODUCTION

CM-I is a common and often debilitating neurologic condition and may result in a variety of signs and symptoms, ranging from headache to brainstem compromise.[1,2] According to some estimates, CM-I is identified in almost 1% of all brain and cervical spine MRI studies,[3,4] although recent evidence suggests that in children the MRI prevalence may be closer to 4%.[5] Although many individuals with radiographic evidence of CM-I are asymptomatic, the clinical manifestations of the disease are broad, complicating efforts to guide patient management and study treatment response. Complicating matters, there is no consensus on the decision to intervene surgically.[6–9] In addition, various investigators have advocated for and against technical variations on foramen magnum decompression with varied opinions but without true experimental conditions.[10]

Assessment of outcomes is complicated by the lack of validated outcome measures specific to CM-I. In recent years, patient-centered approaches to clinical research have become more prominent,[11] and the emphasis on developing and validating rigorous outcome instruments has grown.[12,13] Increasing research efforts in CM-I have focused on comparative effectiveness research[14,15] and on

---

Conflicts of interest and source of funding: The authors do not report any conflicts of interest. The work in this article was not supported by any pertinent funding sources.

[a] Department of Neurological Surgery, Washington University School of Medicine, 660 South Euclid Avenue, Campus Box 8057, St. Louis, MO 63110, USA; [b] Department of Neurological Surgery, St Louis Children's Hospital, Suite 4S20, St Louis, MO 63110, USA

* Corresponding author. Department of Neurological Surgery, Washington University School of Medicine, 660 South Euclid Avenue, Campus Box 8057, St Louis, MO 63110.

E-mail address: yarbroughc@wustl.edu

disease-specific evaluation of clinical outcomes.[16,17] Despite this increased focus on improved research methodology in neurosurgery and other clinical fields, the use of subjective treatment measurement tools remains.[18] This review briefly discusses the various approaches of reporting outcomes in the treatment of patients with CM-I.

The outcome measures reviewed in this article are divided into several broad categories: (1) providing gestalt impression of overall or symptom-specific improvement, (2) using validated quality-of-life (QoL) and disability scores designed to quantify general level of function or disability, (3) using disease-specific, quantifiable methodology to assign numerical scores to symptom status. The first category is largely provider reported, whereas the last 2 categories incorporate patient-centered outcomes. Given the increasing focus on patient-reported outcomes, future studies should consider use of validated patient-centered outcome measures at the expense of gestalt evaluations. For the purposes of this discussion, criterion validity is the concordance of measurements between the instrument and a well-established outcome measure.[19]

GENERAL OUTCOME MEASURES

Before the development of CM-I-specific outcome instruments, many studies used a general gestalt method of determining improvement in clinical status. With minor variations, this method of outcome assessment assigns a patient to improved, stable, or worse categories after therapeutic intervention and has been used in a multitude of case series.[20–26] Although this method of outcome measurement is widely used, it suffers from significant shortfalls. First, the wide variety of symptoms with which patients with CM-I present creates a heterogeneous constellation of symptomatology.[2] Because of the many domains in which symptoms might affect a patient, a simple unidimensional classification scheme does not often suffice to describe fully the change in the clinical signs and symptoms patients with CM-I may face. Second, the signs and symptoms patients experience may affect their outcome differently, a fact not assessed with a simple outcome measure. Third, gestalt impressions do have poor internal or external validity, so comparison of outcomes between or within institutions is problematic when using only this method. Although these limitations are significant, gestalt assessments continue to be used clinically because of convenience and ease of use. A related but more complete method of reporting outcomes includes use of symptom-specific outcomes, although this method also entails use of nonspecific categories similar to the overall gestalt method of outcome assessment.

QUALITY OF LIFE AND DISABILITY SCALES

Because of the absence of robust CM-I-specific measures, some investigators have used general QoL measures not focused on any single disease or have adopted disability scales developed to study conditions other than CM-1 (**Table 1**). Some of these tools focus on evaluation of general

Table 1
General quality-of-life or disability scales used to evaluate clinical outcomes in patients with CM-I

Name of Outcome Tool	Age-group Studied	CM-I Validity	Reliability in CM-I
Euro-Qol-5d[27]	Adults	Yes	No
Headache Disability Index[35]	Adults	No	No
Karnofsky Performance score[28]	Adults & children	No	No
Neck Disability Index[34]	Adults	Yes	No
Noudel et al.'s adapted functional grading system[57]	Adults & children	No	No
Rankin scale[29]	Adults & children	No	No
Short Form-12[30]	Adults	Yes	No
Short Form-36[30]	Adults, unclear if children as well	No	No
Sickness impact profile[31]	Adults & children	No	No
Visual analog scale for disease impact on daily life[32]	Adults & children	No	No
Zung Self-Rating Depression scale[33]	Adults	Yes	No

Adapted from Greenberg JK, Milner E, Yarbrough CK, et al. Outcome methods used in clinical studies of Chiari malformation type I: a systematic review. J Neurosurg 2015;122:265; with permission. Copyright reserved by the American Association of Neurosurgeons.

health and are applicable to a wide range of diseases. For instance, the Euro-Qol-5d,[27] Karnofsky Performance score,[28] Rankin score,[29] SF-12 and SF-36,[30] sickness impact profile,[31] and visual analog scale for disease impact on daily life[32] have each been used in clinical research on CM-I but were designed to measure general QoL and disability rather than specific conditions and outcomes pertinent to CM-I. Each of these has been used once in clinical studies of CM-I.[18]

In addition to such instruments evaluating general function, several tools specifically designed to study diseases such as depression,[33] cervical spine,[34] and headache[35] have been used to assess aspects of common CM-I symptoms quantitatively. Although several of these instruments have criterion validity,[19,36] none of these instruments offer a comprehensive evaluation of the disease-specific outcomes relevant to patients with CM-I. In addition, the validity of Euro-Qol-5d, NDI, SF-12, and Zung Self-Rating Depression scale was assessed in a single study in adult patients.[17]

Although not offering a complete view of CM-I outcomes, several of these general QoL and domain-specific tools have shown criterion validity, that is, concordance with well-established outcome measures, in patients with CM-I.[17] Specifically, NDI and SF-12 show excellent validity for disability and QoL, respectively.[17] These patient-reported outcome measures have been validated in other populations[34,37–39] and can play an important role in quantifying outcomes in CM-I. These measures are briefly described.

Neck Disability Index

The NDI[40] was adapted from 2 earlier measurement tools designed for use in low back pain.[41,42] The NDI (**Table 2**) scores 10 categories, assigning a numerical value from 0 to 5 in each category. Higher scores denote more severe dysfunction. The NDI allows self-rating of disability related to neck pain and has been in wide use.[34] In one study assessing validity of response instruments, the NDI showed the highest criterion validity among several common tools for assessing pain and disability.[17]

Short Form-12

The SF-12[30] is a 12-question instrument designed to evaluate functional status and well-being in 8 health domains. Godil and colleagues[17] demonstrated the validity and responsiveness of the SF-12 physical component scale in assessing general health and QoL in adult patients with CM-I. This assessment tool has the great advantage of widespread use and general acceptance but does not address specific neurologic symptoms or the sequelae of CM-I surgery.

DISEASE-SPECIFIC OUTCOME MEASURES

Several disease-specific instruments have been used to evaluate outcomes in patients with CM-I. See **Table 3** for a listing of the various instruments used. The authors review several widely used and validated instruments in the following discussion.

Japanese Orthopaedic Association Dysfunction Score

The JOA dysfunction score was developed initially in 1975 to assess the functional impairment a patient experiences secondary to myelopathy.[43] This score has been widely used and modified by other investigators (**Table 4**).[44,45] The modified JOA (mJOA) score quantifies dysfunction numerically from 0 to 18, with worse dysfunction signified by lower scores. The mJOA score has been validated in patients with cervical spondylotic myelopathy[46] but not specifically in patients with CM-I. Although this outcome instrument has the advantage of assessing motor and sensory deficits attributable to cervical spinal cord pathology, it does not fully address other problematic aspects of CM-I symptomatology, such as headache, cranial nerve dysfunction, and complications related to surgical intervention.

Asgari Score

The Asgari score[47] was developed specifically for syringomyelia related to hindbrain disorders and has undergone modifications to increase its relevance to patients with CM-I (**Table 5**).[48,49] This outcome instrument scores 2 different components: cranial nerve involvement and spinal cord dysfunction. This scoring system was initially developed to evaluate dysfunction secondary to syringomyelia, thus leading to a focus on cervical spinal cord dysfunction. The spinal cord is evaluated both with respect to upper extremity function and lower extremity function with respect to walking. A score from 1 to 10 is possible, with 1 to 3 denoting slight, 4 to 6 moderate, and 7 to 10 severe dysfunction. This scale provides a detailed evaluation of the functional disability related to cervical spinal cord disease but is intended for retrospective chart review rather than patient-defined assessments. In addition, it has not been validated in patients with CM-1.

Chicago Chiari Outcome Score

In response to some of the shortcomings outlined for previous outcome measures, the CCOS was

Table 2
The Neck Disability Index

Characteristic	0	1	2	3	4	5
				Score		
Pain	No pain	Very mild	Moderate	Fairly severe	Very severe	Worst imaginable
Personal care (washing, dressing)	No limits	No limits but causes pain	Painful, slow and careful	Requires some help, but can manage most care	Requires help every day in most aspects	Cannot get dressed, washes with difficulty, stays in bed
Lifting	Heavy weights without pain	Heavy weights with pain	Limited with heavy weights, cannot pick up off floor	Pain prevents lifting heavy weights but can manage light weights	Can lift very light weights only	Cannot lift anything
Reading	Unlimited	Unlimited with slight pain in neck	Unlimited with moderate pain	Limited because of moderate neck pain	Difficulty reading because of severe pain	Cannot read because of pain
Headaches	None	Slight, infrequent	Moderate, infrequent	Moderate, frequent	Severe, frequent	Nearly constant
Concentration	Full without limits	Full with slight difficulty	Fair difficulty	A lot of difficulty	Great difficulty	Cannot concentrate
Work	Unlimited	Only usual work	Most of usual work	Cannot do usual work	Hardly any work	Cannot work
Driving	Can drive without any pain	Can drive with slight pain	Can drive with moderate pain	Cannot drive because of moderate pain	Can hardly drive because of severe pain	Cannot drive
Sleeping	No trouble	Slight disturbance (<1 h sleepless)	Mild disturbance (1–2 h sleepless)	Moderate disturbance (2–3 h sleepless)	Great disturbance (3–5 h sleepless)	Complete disturbance (5–7 h sleepless)
Recreation	Can perform all activities	All activities with some pain	Most activities, limited by neck pain	A few of normal activities, limited by neck pain	Hardly any recreation because of neck pain	No recreational activities

Adapted from Vernon H, Mior S. The neck disability index: a study of reliability and validity. J Manipulative Physiol Ther 1991;14(7):411; with permission.

Table 3
Disease-specific scales used to evaluate clinical outcomes in patients treated for CM-I

Name of Outcome Tool	Age-group Studied	CM-I Validity	Reliability in CM-I
Asgari score (modified)[48,49]	Adults	No	No
Chicago Chiari Outcome Scale[16]	Adults & children	Yes	Yes
Japanese Orthopaedic Association score[43,45]	Adults & children	No	No
Klekamp & Samii score[51,52,58]	Adults & children	No	No
Limonadi score[59]	Adults & children	No	No
Visual analog score-pain[60]	Adults	No	No

Adapted from Greenberg JK, Milner E, Yarbrough CK, et al. Outcome methods used in clinical studies of Chiari malformation type I: a systematic review. J Neurosurg 2015;122:265; with permission. Copyright reserved by the American Association of Neurosurgeons.

developed and internally validated (**Table 6**).[16] The CCOS was subsequently validated in an external sample in the pediatric population.[50] This measurement instrument quantitatively evaluates improvement in pain and nonpain domains, along with general impairment of functional status. The CCOS also introduces an evaluation of operative complications, although the specific subscores

Table 4
The Japanese Orthopaedic Association score for cervical myelopathy

	Definition
Motor Dysfunction of Upper Extremities	
0	Inability to move hands
1	Inability to eat with a spoon but able to use hands
2	Inability to button shirt but able to eat with a spoon
3	Able to button shirt with great difficulty
4	Able to button shirt with slight difficulty
5	No dysfunction
Motor Dysfunction of Lower Extremities	
0	Complete loss of motor and sensory function
1	Sensory preservation without ability to move legs
2	Able to move legs but unable to walk
3	Able to walk on flat floor with a walking aid
4	Able to walk up and down stairs with a handrail
5	Moderate to significant lack of stability but able to walk up and down stairs without handrail
6	Mild lack of stability but able to walk with smooth reciprocation unaided
7	No dysfunction
Sensory Dysfunction of Upper Extremities	
0	Complete loss of hand sensation
1	Severe sensory loss or pain
2	Mild sensory loss
3	No sensory loss
Sphincter Dysfunction Score	
0	Inability to micturate voluntarily
1	Marked difficulty with urination
2	Mild to moderate difficulty with micturition
3	Normal micturition

From Benzel EC, Lancon J, Kesterson L, et al. Cervical laminectomy and dentate ligament section for cervical spondylotic myelopathy. J Spinal Disord 1991;4(3):289; with permission.

Table 5
The Asgari scoring system

Score	Finding
Cranial nerves	
2	Cranial nerve involvement
Upper extremities	
2	Moderate disability in upper extremities
3	Complete disability in upper extremities
Lower extremities	
1	Spinal cord signs but no difficulty walking
2	Slight difficulty with upper and/or lower extremities that does not prevent full-time employment
3	Difficulty walking that prevents full-time employment or ability to perform housework but can walk without assistance
4	Can walk only with help or a frame
5	Cannot walk

This scoring system scores cranial nerve involvement, upper extremity disability, and lower extremity function to quantify neurologic dysfunction.

From Asgari S, Engelhorn T, Bschor M, et al. Surgical prognosis in hindbrain related syringomyelia. Acta Neurol Scand 2003;107(1):14; with permission.

are somewhat ambiguous. In the external validation of the CCOS, the reliability of the functionality subscore was poor.[50] This poor reliability largely resulted from divergent interpretation of the differences between subscores 2 and 3 and between subscores 3 and 4 (see **Table 3**). Another shortcoming of the CCOS is that there are few patients with a poor outcome, leading to a clustering of CCOS scores at the high end of the spectrum. Thus, although the CCOS has performed well in evaluating patients with CM-I via retrospective chart review, there are some weaknesses that must be considered when using it to compare CM-I treatment results.

Table 6
Chicago Chiari Outcome Scale

Characteristic	Score			
	1	**2**	**3**	**4**
Pain	Worse	Unchanged and refractory to medication	Improved or controlled with medication	Resolved
Nonpain	Worse	Unchanged or improved but impaired	Improved and unimpaired	Resolved
Functionality	Unable to attend	Moderate impairment (<50% attendance)	Mild impairment (>50% attendance)	Fully functional
Complication	Persistent complication, poorly controlled	Persistent complication, well controlled	Transient complication	Uncomplicated course

Details of the CCOS as reported in Aliaga L, Hekman KE, Yassari R, et al. A novel scoring system for assessing Chiari malformation type I treatment outcomes. Neurosurgery 2012;70(3):656–64. [discussion: 664–5].

Adapted from Yarbrough CK, Greenberg JK, Smyth MD, et al. External validation of the Chicago Chiari Outcome Scale. J Neurosurg Pediatr. 2014;13(6):680; with permission. Copyright reserved by the American Association of Neurosurgeons.

Klekamp and Samii Score

Klekamp and Samii[51] developed a numeric scale evaluating spinal cord dysfunction in several domains. This score was subsequently updated and has been used to evaluate outcomes in a large case series of patients with CM-I.[52] The Klekamp and Samii score targets pain, sensory changes, motor function, ataxia, urinary difficulty, and swallowing function. Each domain is scored similarly: 0, no function; 1, severely disabled; 2, disabled; 3, severely compromised but function preserved; 4, slightly compromised; 5, normal function. Similar to the Asgari score and mJOA, the Klekamp and Samii score focuses on dysfunction secondary to spine pathology and thus does not evaluate headache, neck pain, or functional outcomes.

Chiari Symptom Profile

Mueller and Oro[53] have developed a patient-reported outcome instrument specific for patients with CM-I with high validity and reliability when tested internally. The Chiari Symptom Profile uses a rating scale from 0 to 4 on each of 57 questions, for a possible numeric score ranging from 0 (no disability) to 228 (severe disability). This scoring system requires a significant time investment from each patient but has shown promise for use in outcomes research. Nonetheless, external validation and further demonstrations of practical usability in clinical studies are needed to firmly establish the role of the Chiari Symptom Profile in CM-I research.

DISCUSSION

The earlier discussion details the variety of approaches used to evaluate the treatment of patients with CM-I. A recent systematic review discusses these strategies and their use in more detail.[18] Using consistent outcome instruments with high interrater reliability should be encouraged and is necessary to develop evidence-based treatment algorithms. The patient experience in CM-I is variable, increasing the challenge to clinical researchers to evaluate treatment algorithms among different institutions.

The adoption of general QoL and disability scales from other fields has led to increasing emphasis on defining clinical outcomes from the patient's view (eg, patient-defined outcomes), rather than the simplified view of gestalt evaluation. Although many general scales are available, the NDI, Euro-QoL-5d, and SF-12 physical component scale have shown the highest validity in patients with CM-I.[17] The use of these scales

allows quantification of QoL and allows for conversion of scores to utilities for cost-utility analysis.[17,54] In the absence of a specific, validated QOL instrument designed for patients with CM-I, inclusion of at least 1 of these scales for determination of patient QoL is recommended for clinical research involving patients with CM-I.

Increasing sophistication in clinical research has led to development of several disease-specific outcome instruments that have been validated for use in studies. Although most of the instruments discussed earlier were initially developed to evaluate spine pathology, the CCOS stands out as a tool developed specifically to study CM-I (see **Table 3**). This measure has been validated in adult and pediatric patients[16,50] and has been used in multiple clinical studies.[17,50,55,56] However, it has several key weaknesses, including poor interrater reliability of the functionality subscore and a reliance on retrospective chart review rather than patient-defined impressions.[50] The recently developed Chiari Symptom Profile has shown strong internal validity[53] but must be externally validated and used in additional studies to establish its role in outcomes research.

The inherent variability of the patient experience in CM-I requires the implementation of patient-centered outcome instruments to adequately assess the symptoms of CM-I. The development of validated outcome instruments obligates the inclusion of the patient-defined experience in assessment of treatment strategies in the future.

SUMMARY

Investigators have used several strategies to evaluate patients with CM-I, from a general gestalt impression of outcome to validated patient-reported outcome measures. Although no scale is complete in all respects, the NDI and SF-12 have excellent validity to assess general QoL and function in the CM-I population. The development of the CCOS allows some quantification of the often complex postoperative course patients experience. Further refinement and increased use of these validated outcome scales should be encouraged and will lead to easier comparison of treatment strategies.

REFERENCES

1. Aitken LA, Lindan CE, Sidney S, et al. Chiari type I malformation in a pediatric population. Pediatr Neurol 2009;40(6):449–54.
2. Milhorat TH, Chou MW, Trinidad EM, et al. Chiari I malformation redefined: clinical and radiographic

findings for 364 symptomatic patients. Neurosurgery 1999;44(5):1005–17.

3. Meadows J, Kraut M, Guarnieri M, et al. Asymptomatic Chiari type I malformations identified on magnetic resonance imaging. J Neurosurg 2000;92(6):920–6.

4. Smith BW, Strahle J, Bapuraj JR, et al. Distribution of cerebellar tonsil position: implications for understanding Chiari malformation. J Neurosurg 2013; 119(3):812–9.

5. Strahle J, Muraszko KM, Kapurch J, et al. Chiari malformation type I and syrinx in children undergoing magnetic resonance imaging. J Neurosurg Pediatr 2011;8(2):205–13.

6. Caldarelli M, Novegno F, Vassimi L, et al. The role of limited posterior fossa craniectomy in the surgical treatment of Chiari malformation type I: experience with a pediatric series. J Neurosurg 2007;106(3 Suppl):187–95.

7. Di X. Endoscopic suboccipital decompression on pediatric Chiari type I. Minim Invasive Neurosurg 2009;52(3):119–25.

8. Erdogan E, Cansever T, Secer HI, et al. The evaluation of surgical treatment options in the Chiari malformation type I. Turk Neurosurg 2010;20(3):303–13.

9. Parker SR, Harris P, Cummings TJ, et al. Complications following decompression of Chiari malformation type I in children: dural graft or sealant? J Neurosurg Pediatr 2011;8(2):177–83.

10. Alden TD, Ojemann JG, Park TS. Surgical treatment of Chiari I malformation: indications and approaches. Neurosurg Focus 2001;11(1):E2.

11. Selby JV, Beal AC, Frank L. The Patient-Centered Outcomes Research Institute (PCORI) national priorities for research and initial research agenda. JAMA 2012;307(15):1583–4.

12. Mokkink LB, Terwee CB, Patrick DL, et al. The COSMIN study reached international consensus on taxonomy, terminology, and definitions of measurement properties for health-related patient-reported outcomes. J Clin Epidemiol 2010;63(7):737–45.

13. Mokkink LB, Terwee CB, Patrick DL, et al. The COSMIN checklist for assessing the methodological quality of studies on measurement properties of health status measurement instruments: an international Delphi study. Qual Life Res 2010;19(4):539–49.

14. Durham SR, Fjeld-Olenec K. Comparison of posterior fossa decompression with and without duraplasty for the surgical treatment of Chiari malformation type I in pediatric patients: a meta-analysis. J Neurosurg Pediatr 2008;2(1):42–9.

15. Hankinson T, Tubbs RS, Wellons JC. Duraplasty or not? An evidence-based review of the pediatric Chiari I malformation. Childs Nerv Syst 2011;27(1):35–40.

16. Aliaga L, Hekman KE, Yassari R, et al. A novel scoring system for assessing Chiari malformation type I treatment outcomes. Neurosurgery 2012; 70(3):656–64 [discussion: 664–5].

17. Godil SS, Parker SL, Zuckerman SL, et al. Accurately measuring outcomes after surgery for adult Chiari I malformation: determining the most valid and responsive instruments. Neurosurgery 2013;72(5):820–7.

18. Greenberg JK, Milner E, Yarbrough CK, et al. Outcome methods used in clinical studies of Chiari malformation type I: a systematic review. J Neurosurg 2014;122:1–11.

19. Hulley SB, Cummings SR, Browner WS, et al. Designing clinical research. 3rd edition. Philadelphia: Lippincott Williams & Wilkins; 2007.

20. Alzate JC, Kothbauer KF, Jallo GI, et al. Treatment of Chiari I malformation in patients with and without syringomyelia: a consecutive series of 66 cases. Neurosurg Focus 2001;11(1):E3.

21. Galarza M, Sood S, Ham S. Relevance of surgical strategies for the management of pediatric Chiari type I malformation. Childs Nerv Syst 2007;23(6):691–6.

22. Navarro R, Olavarria G, Seshadri R, et al. Surgical results of posterior fossa decompression for patients with Chiari I malformation. Childs Nerv Syst 2004; 20(5):349–56.

23. Tubbs RS, Beckman J, Naftel RP, et al. Institutional experience with 500 cases of surgically treated pediatric Chiari malformation type I. J Neurosurg Pediatr 2011;7(3):248–56.

24. Ventureyra EC, Aziz HA, Vassilyadi M. The role of cine flow MRI in children with Chiari I malformation. Childs Nerv Syst 2003;19(2):109–13.

25. Yarbrough CK, Powers AK, Park TS, et al. Patients with Chiari malformation type I presenting with acute neurological deficits: case series. J Neurosurg Pediatr 2011;7(3):244–7.

26. Paul KS, Lye RH, Strang FA, et al. Arnold-Chiari malformation. Review of 71 cases. J Neurosurg 1983; 58(2):183–7.

27. EuroQol-Group. EQ-5D. Available at: http://www.euroqol.org/home.html. Accessed November 1, 2013.

28. Yates JW, Chalmer B, McKegney FP. Evaluation of patients with advanced cancer using the Karnofsky performance status. Cancer 1980;45(8):2220–4.

29. Lai SM, Duncan PW. Evaluation of the American Heart Association Stroke Outcome Classification. Stroke 1999;30(9):1840–3.

30. QualityMetric. SF Health Surveys. 2013. Available at: http://www.qualitymetric.com/WhatWeDo/SFHealthSurveys/tabid/184/Default.aspx. Accessed January 14, 2015.

31. Mueller D, Oro JJ. Prospective analysis of self-perceived quality of life before and after posterior fossa decompression in 112 patients with Chiari malformation with or without syringomyelia. Neurosurg Focus 2005;18(2):ECP2.

32. Tisell M, Wallskog J, Linde M. Long-term outcome after surgery for Chiari I malformation. Acta Neurol Scand 2009;120(5):295–9.

33. Zung WW, Richards CB, Short MJ. Self-rating depression scale in an outpatient clinic. Further

validation of the SDS. Arch Gen Psychiatry 1965; 13(6):508–15.

34. Vernon H. The neck disability index: state-of-the-art, 1991–2008. J Manipulative Physiol Ther 2008;31(7): 491–502.

35. Pryse-Phillips W. Evaluating migraine disability: the headache impact test instrument in context. Can J Neurol Sci 2002;29(Suppl 2):S11–5.

36. Carmines EG, Zeller RA. Reliability and validity assessment, vol. 17. Newbury Park (CA): Sage Publications Inc; 1979.

37. Usai S, Grazzi L, D'Amico D, et al. Psychological variables in chronic migraine with medication overuse before and after inpatient withdrawal: results at 1-year follow-up. Neurol Sci 2009;30(Suppl 1):S125–7.

38. Lipton RB, Hamelsky SW, Kolodner KB, et al. Migraine, quality of life, and depression: a population-based case-control study. Neurology 2000;55(5):629–35.

39. Carreon LY, Glassman SD, Campbell MJ, et al. Neck Disability Index, short form-36 physical component summary, and pain scales for neck and arm pain: the minimum clinically important difference and substantial clinical benefit after cervical spine fusion. Spine J 2010;10(6):469–74.

40. Vernon H, Mior S. The Neck Disability Index: a study of reliability and validity. J Manipulative Physiol Ther 1991;14(7):409–15.

41. Roland M, Morris R. A study of the natural history of back pain. Part I: development of a reliable and sensitive measure of disability in low-back pain. Spine 1983;8(2):141–4.

42. Fairbank JC, Couper J, Davies JB, et al. The Oswestry low back pain disability questionnaire. Physiotherapy 1980;66(8):271–3.

43. Fukui M, Chiba K, Kawakami M, et al. An outcome measure for patients with cervical myelopathy: Japanese Orthopaedic Association Cervical Myelopathy Evaluation Questionnaire (JOACMEQ): part 1. J Orthop Sci 2007;12(3):227–40.

44. Benzel EC, Lancon J, Kesterson L, et al. Cervical laminectomy and dentate ligament section for cervical spondylotic myelopathy. J Spinal Disord 1991; 4(3):286–95.

45. Yilmaz A, Kanat A, Musluman AM, et al. When is duraplasty required in the surgical treatment of Chiari malformation type I based on tonsillar descending grading scale? World Neurosurg 2011; 75(2):307–13.

46. Yonenobu K, Abumi K, Nagata K, et al. Interobserver and intraobserver reliability of the Japanese Orthopaedic Association scoring system for evaluation of cervical compression myelopathy. Spine 2001; 26(17):1890–4 [discussion: 1895].

47. Asgari S, Engelhorn T, Bschor M, et al. Surgical prognosis in hindbrain related syringomyelia. Acta Neurol Scand 2003;107(1):12–21.

48. Koc K, Anik Y, Anik I, et al. Chiari 1 malformation with syringomyelia: correlation of phase-contrast cine MR imaging and outcome. Turk Neurosurg 2007; 17(3):183–92.

49. Furtado SV, Thakar S, Hegde AS. Correlation of functional outcome and natural history with clinicoradiological factors in surgically managed pediatric Chiari I malformation. Neurosurgery 2011;68(2): 319–27 [discussion: 328].

50. Yarbrough CK, Greenberg JK, Smyth MD, et al. External validation of the Chicago Chiari Outcome Scale. J Neurosurg Pediatr 2014;13(6):679–84.

51. Klekamp J, Samii M. Introduction of a score system for the clinical evaluation of patients with spinal processes. Acta Neurochir (Wein) 1993;123(3–4): 221–3.

52. Klekamp J. Surgical treatment of Chiari I malformation – analysis of intraoperative findings, complications, and outcome for 371 foramen magnum decompressions. Neurosurgery 2012;71(2):365–80 [discussion: 380].

53. Mueller DM, Oro JJ. The Chiari Symptom Profile: development and validation of a Chiari-/syringomyelia-specific questionnaire. J Neurosci Nurs 2013; 45(4):205–10.

54. Richardson SS, Berven S. The development of a model for translation of the Neck Disability Index to utility scores for cost-utility analysis in cervical disorders. Spine J 2012;12(1):55–62.

55. Lee A, Yarbrough CK, Greenberg JK, et al. Comparison of posterior fossa decompression with or without duraplasty in children with type I Chiari malformation. Childs Nerv Syst 2014;30(8):1419–24.

56. Hekman KE, Aliaga L, Straus D, et al. Positive and negative predictors for good outcome after decompressive surgery for Chiari malformation type 1 as scored on the Chicago Chiari Outcome Scale. Neurol Res 2012;34(7):694–700.

57. Noudel R, Gomis P, Sotoares G, et al. Posterior fossa volume increase after surgery for Chiari malformation type I: a quantitative assessment using magnetic resonance imaging and correlations with the treatment response. J Neurosurg 2011;115(3):647–58.

58. Arora P, Pradhan PK, Behari S, et al. Chiari I malformation related syringomyelia: radionuclide cisternography as a predictor of outcome. Acta Neurochir (Wein) 2004;146(2):119–30.

59. Limonadi FM, Selden NR. Dura-splitting decompression of the craniocervical junction: reduced operative time, hospital stay, and cost with equivalent early outcome. J Neurosurg 2004;101(2 Suppl): 184–8.

60. Ono A, Numasawa T, Wada K, et al. Surgical outcomes of foramen magnum decompression for syringomyelia associated with Chiari I malformation: relation between the location of the syrinx and body pain. J Orthop Sci 2010;15(3):299–304.

Surgical History of Sleep Apnea in Pediatric Patients with Chiari Type 1 Malformation

Isaac Jonathan Pomeraniec, BSc, Alexander Ksendzovsky, MD,
Pearl L. Yu, MD, John A. Jane Jr, MD*

KEYWORDS

- Chiari malformation • Sleep apnea • Duraplasty • Dural splitting

KEY POINTS

- Sleep apnea represents a relative indication for posterior fossa decompression (PFD) in pediatric patients with Chiari malformation type 1 (CM-1).
- Duraplasty was associated with improvement of sleep apnea in 100% of patients and dural splitting with improvement in 50% of patients.
- Duraplasty and dural splitting were associated with a similar reduction in tonsillar herniation on radiographic imaging of 58% (37% excluding tonsillectomy) and 35%, respectively.
- Intraoperative ultrasound can be beneficial in determining restoration of cerebrospinal fluid (CSF) circulation in the posterior fossa.
- Longitudinal follow-up studies of patients with either neurologic deficits or severe symptoms will further elucidate the natural history of CM-1 and more appropriately gauge the risk-benefit tradeoff of surgical intervention.

Videos of tonsillopexy, dural splitting technique, and intraoperative ultrasound showing visualization of underlying tonsils accompany this article at http://www.neurosurgery.theclinics.com/.

INTRODUCTION

CM-1 has become increasingly recognized as a significant clinical burden in approximately 3.6% of children undergoing brain and cervical spinal cord imaging.[1,2] Although approximately two-thirds of children are asymptomatic and present with incidental findings, symptoms can result from compression of neural structures in the posterior fossa and be associated with syrinx of the spinal cord or brainstem.[3,4] Children can also have more occult findings, such as ataxia, sensory and motor deficits, lower cranial nerve abnormalities, or merely irritability or neck arching.[5]

The association between Chiari-related herniation and sleep apnea syndromes is described elsewhere.[6–10] Although sleep apnea syndromes are rare in childhood, with a prevalence of approximately 1% to 3%, recent series have reported upwards of 60% in children with CM-1.[11–14] Sleep-related breathing disruption results from compression of the medullary respiratory control centers

Department of Neurological Surgery, University of Virginia Health Science Center, 1215 Lee Street, Charlottesville, VA 22908, USA
* Corresponding author. Department of Neurological Surgery, University of Virginia Health Science Center, PO Box 800212, Charlottesville, VA 22908-0711, USA.
E-mail address: jaj2k@virginia.edu

Neurosurg Clin N Am 26 (2015) 543–553
http://dx.doi.org/10.1016/j.nec.2015.06.009
1042-3680/15/$ – see front matter © 2015 Elsevier Inc. All rights reserved.

and manifests in central or obstructive sleep apnea, hypoventilation, or even sudden death.[14–19] Brainstem compression in addition to strain on lower cranial nerves may also result in dysphagia, hoarseness of voice with decreased vocal cord mobility, dysarthria, palatal and hypoglossal weakness, and recurrent aspiration.[20] Although surgical decompression serves as the preferred treatment of sleep-disordered breathing in patients with Chiari malformation, the effect of surgery differs among patients and respiratory failure can be a complication of treatment.[6,8,9,21–26] Reports have proposed not only increased incidence of respiratory arrest and death during sleep but also nocturnal respiratory depression during the immediate postoperative period (up to 14% of patients in the first 5 days), presumably secondary to edema formation.[6,21,22,27]

Without a widely recognized, definitive correlation between magnitude of tonsillar herniation and clinical manifestations of cervicomedullary junction compression, debate lingers over the indications for operative versus nonoperative management of CM-1.[5,28–32] As such, there are no generally accepted criteria for selecting patients with CM-1 for surgical treatment and the decision for suboccipital decompression for symptomatic relief can be subjective.[20] A recent review by the current authors (Pomeraniec, Ksendzovksy, Jane Jr, personal communication, 2015.) of 95 consecutive cases of Chiari type 1 malformation in pediatric patients identified dysphagia and sleep apnea as symptoms indicating surgical management.

The purpose of this review is 2-fold: (1) review the long-term clinical and radiographic information for surgically managed pediatric patients with concurrent sleep apnea and CM-1 and (2) review the literature and provide a representative case series comparing 2 different surgical techniques (duraplasty and dural splitting) as well as their correlation to symptomatic and radiographic resolution or progression.

METHODS

The authors retrospectively reviewed 8 consecutive pediatric patients (less than 18 years old) with suspected symptomatic sleep apnea and concurrent CM-1 (defined as herniation of the cerebellar tonsils at least 5 mm below the foramen magnum) who were treated at the University of Virginia between 2004 and 2014. One patient was treated conservatively and followed in the outpatient setting. Seven patients received PFD and were grouped based on operative technique: 3 patients underwent duraplasty (1 with tonsillectomy, 1 with tonsillopexy, and 1 with tonsils untouched) and 4 patients underwent a dural splitting technique.

Clinical Evaluation

Patients underwent comprehensive multidisciplinary evaluation, including child neurology, sleep specialist, and otolaryngology consultations with information available about history, neurologic examinations, polysomnography data, vocal cord mobility, upper airway motor dysfunction, and swallowing difficulty. The patients were treated/operated on by the same pediatric neurosurgeon.

Imaging

All patients underwent high-resolution MRI using standard T1- and T2-weighted spin-echo sequences. Imaging studies were independently reviewed at diagnosis by a neuroradiologist and pediatric neurosurgeon for amount of cerebellar tonsillar ectopia, CSF flow dynamics at the foramen magnum, and spinal cord syringomyelia. The authors defined a syrinx as a contiguous fluid collection (hypointense on T1-weighted images with corresponding T2 hyperintensity) of at least 2 mm in maximal anteroposterior diameter on sagittal or axial imaging suggesting fluid within the spinal cord. If a syrinx was present, its widest diameter in millimeters as viewed on sagittal imaging and its length according to number of spanning vertebral levels were reported. Presyrinx states (T2 hyperintensity with indistinct T1 prolongation and without cavitation) were separately classified. CSF flow at the foramen magnum was evaluated by cine MRI. Sagittal CSF flow studies at the craniocervical junction were evaluated for CSF pulsations across the anterior and posterior midline foramen magnum as well as for any abnormally exaggerated cranial or caudal pulsations of the lower brainstem, upper cervical cord, or cerebellar tonsils. Baseline imaging parameters were compared with findings on postoperative imaging.

Sleep Evaluation

Patients were evaluated in the University of Virginia Sleep Disorders Laboratory. Standard testing consisted of electroencephalogram (C3/A2, C2/A1, O1/A2, and O2/A1), electromyogram (chin), electro-oculography (right/left), ECG, oxygen saturation by digital pulse oximetry, nasal/oral airflow by thermistor or nasal pressure cannula, end-tidal CO_2 by nasal cannula, and qualitative thoracic/abdominal movement by respiratory inductive plethysmography. Natural sleep was observed overnight. No sedation was administered. Central apneas, obstructive apneas, hypopneas, periodic breathing, the adequacy of gas exchange, and heart rate were recorded during sleep.

Surgical Technique

For patients undergoing PFD, a midline incision was made from the inion to the C2 level and carried down the midline using sharp dissection through the midline raphe to expose the suboccipital region of C1 and upper portion of C2. A suboccipital craniectomy was performed with a high-speed drill (**Fig. 1**A) with the foramen magnum decompression measuring a minimum of 2 cm wide and 2 cm above the foramen (see **Fig. 1**B, C). C1 laminectomy was performed in all patients and a C2 laminectomy was performed in those patients whose tonsils extended to that level. Intraoperative ultrasound was performed before and after duraplasty and/or dural splitting but in no case was a planned dural splitting technique converted to a duraplasty on the basis of ultrasound. For duraplasty cases, arachnoid adhesions were released with sharp dissection and tonsillar coagulation or tonsillar resection was performed if these techniques were judged necessary to restore normal 4th ventricular CSF outflow. Duraplasty was performed using collagen-based dural substitutes. For those who underwent dural splitting, the superficial layer of the dura was split and opened without completely cutting through the inferior layer until the dura was translucent. The dural band at the foramen magnum was released.

Duraplasty

Under microscope visualization, a Woodson elevator was used to elevate the thick and tense band constituting the outer leaf of the foramen magnum dura and periosteum, which was encountered invariably in all patients (**Fig. 2**). With thinning of the dural band, there was a subsequent release of pressure at the cervicomedullary junction, giving more room for expansion of herniated cerebellar tonsils, which were visualized pulsating under the microscope. The dura was then incised in a Y-shape under the microscope and held open by sutures tacked laterally and superiorly. The arachnoid

was inspected for any scarring and adhesions, which were sharply dissected if present, and the thick band of arachnoid between the tonsils and dura was sharply released. For tonsillectomy (n = 1), dissection was taken circumferentially around the tonsils, which were subsequently elevated with careful dissection from underneath C2. The inferior portion of the tonsils were cauterized, incised and internally debulked. For tonsillopexy (n = 1) (Video 1; available online at http://www.neurosurgery.theclinics.com/), tonsils were mobilized from below the level of the dural opening and subsequently cauterized superiorly with bipolar electrocautery. For duraplasty with tonsils untouched (n = 1), the tonsils themselves were not scarred down and an easy dissection was taken between and beneath the tonsils. A fashioned piece of artificial dura (Duragen [Medtronic] or Durepair [Integra]) was used for the duraplasty and tacked into place. A central tacking suture was placed in the dural graft through the fascia or muscle to avoid adherence of the dural graft to underlying arachnoid. The dural graft was covered with DuraSeal (in 1 patient) or gel foam and the closure was performed in standard layered fashion. All patients were admitted to the neurosurgical ICU postoperatively.

Dural Splitting

Adherent fibers between the posterior atlantooccipital membrane and dura were similarly removed and the fibrous band was released sharply (**Fig. 3**). Once the thick fibrous band was incised, a dissector was used to split the dura caudally and laterally to the inferior and lateral extent of the bony exposure. A vertical incision was made of the outer layer of the dura, laterally from the midline. Using blunt dissection the outer layer of the dura was removed without breaching the inner layer or the arachnoid membrane. The cerebellar tonsils were then easily seen pulsating through the thinned dura (Video 2; available online at http://www.neurosurgery.theclinics.com/). The

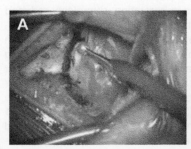
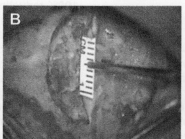
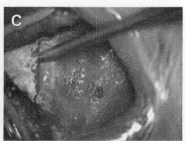

Fig. 1. Suboccipital craniectomy. (*A–C*) Bone removal of the foramen magnum. Foramen magnum decompression was performed measuring a minimum of 2 cm wide and 2 cm above the foramen.

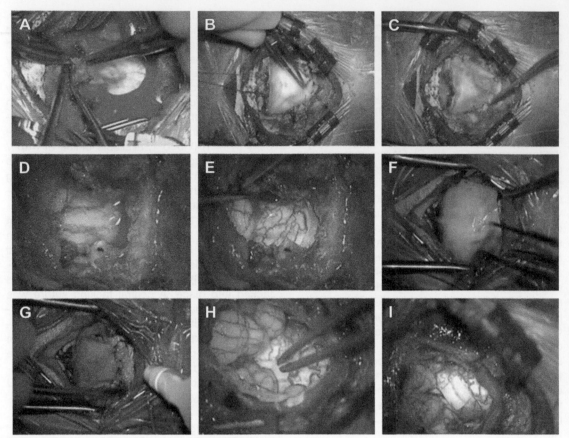

Fig. 2. Duraplasty. (*A*) Removal of thick fibrous dural band. (*B, C*) Dural tack-up suture. (*D, E*) Open arachnoid, no adhesions. (*F, G*) Duraplasty. (*H, I*) Tonsillopexy.

ultrasound was used to visualize the tonsils, which were seen to move freely (Video 3; available online at http://www.neurosurgery.theclinics.com/). CSF was identified posterior to the tonsils and between the dura as well as below the inferior aspect of the tonsils. The tonsils, which had been compressed and were pointed preoperatively, had been obviously freed and had a much more rounded appearance, indicating their decompression. The dura appeared transparent and bluish. Muscular and subcutaneous planes were closed without any tension.

RESULTS
Patient Characteristics

In total, 8 pediatric patients were evaluated for and diagnosed with CM-1 and attendant central sleep apnea. One patient was treated conservatively without surgery and 7 patients received PFD with either duraplasty (n = 3) or dural splitting (n = 4). The average age at presentation was 11.9 years (range 2.2–17.1 years). Median clinical follow-up was 47.4 months (range 3.2–98.3 months) and

median imaging follow-up was 45.7 months (range 3.2–107.4 months).

Imaging Characteristics

The mean extent of tonsillar herniation below foramen magnum at presentation was 22.2 mm (range 9.5–37.0 mm). Across all surgical patients, preoperative tonsillar descent ranged from 14.0 to 37.0 mm. On average, duraplasty reduced tonsillar herniation by 58% and dural splitting by 35%. Excluding the 1 patient with tonsillectomy and 100% reduction in herniation, duraplasty reduced tonsillar herniation by 37%. There was no significant difference of reduction in tonsillar herniation between duraplasty (16.2 mm) and dural splitting (9.7 mm, average) (*P* = .40), which was further elucidated when excluding the patient who underwent tonsillectomy (*P* = .92) (**Table 1**).

One patient (33%) in the duraplasty group and 1 patient (25%) In the dural splitting group presented with syrinx. One patient in the duraplasty (tonsillopexy) group developed syrinx after the first decompression, which resolved with repeat

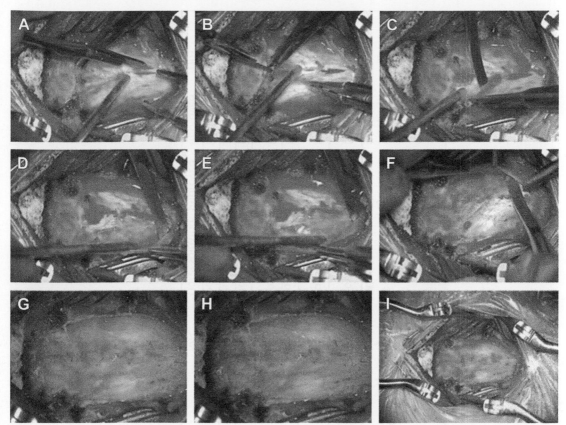

Fig. 3. Dural splitting. For those who underwent dural splitting, the superficial layer of the dura was split and opened without completely cutting through the inferior layer until the dura was translucent. (*A*) Incising the dura. (*B*) Splitting the dural band at the foramen magnum. (*C–F*) Bluntly dissecting between the leaves of the dura and then sharply dividing perpendicularly to periosteal fibers. (*G, H*) Thinned dura. (*I*) Final thinned dura.

tonsillopexy and reconstruction of the subarachnoid space. All patients with a syrinx had at least 1 repeat MRI study of the spine. These repeat imaging studies revealed resolution of syrinx size (eg, no evidence of syringomyelia on postoperative MRI) in both patients with surgery. Two patients (50%) in the dural splitting group developed presyrinx before surgery and both of these patients exhibited resolution of presyrinx after surgery (**Table 2**).

Table 1
Tonsillar descent below foramen magnum

	Below, Average (mm)	Below, Most Recent (mm)	Difference, Average, mm (% Change)
Nonsurgical	9.5	15.5	6.0 (63)
Duraplasty	23.0	6.7	−16.2 (−58)
Dural splitting	24.8	18.6	−9.7 (−35)

Clinical Characteristics

All 8 patients experienced central sleep apnea related to CM-1. One patient in the dural splitting group experienced both central and obstructive sleep apnea. The 1 patient who was managed conservatively was diagnosed with CM-1 as an incident finding during work-up for seizures. Only 1 patient (in the dural splitting group) had no additional symptoms. In total, 6 patients also presented with headache: 3 of 4 patients (75%) in both the duraplasty and dural splitting groups. Other symptoms included sensorimotor (n = 3), visual (n = 1), and dysphagia (n = 1). All 7 surgical patients (100%) experienced improvement in these symptoms over the follow-up period ($P = 1.00$). Based on number of central and obstructive apnea episodes and hypopneas during sleep studies, only 5 (62.5%) surgical patients experienced improvement of sleep apnea whereas the remaining 2 (37.5%) experienced no change. All 3 patients (100%) in the duraplasty group experienced improved sleep apnea versus 2 of 4 (50%) patients in the dural splitting group, although this

Table 2
Clinical presentation and follow-up

Age[a] (Surgery), Gender	Follow-up Length,[b] (Clinical)	Follow-up Length,[b] (Imaging)	Neurologic Examination	Other Symptoms (in Addition to Sleep Apnea)	Syrinx Level	Management	Symptom Course	Sleep Apnea Course	Syrinx Course
2.2[c] M	53.0	49.5	Delayed language	Incidental[d]	N/A	Conservative	No change	No change	N/A
16.4 M	68.1	68.1	Nystagmus, Romberg	H/A, motor	C3	Tonsillectomy	Improved	Improved	Resolved
12.9 F	98.3	107.4	Normal	H/A, visual, sensory	N/A	Tonsillopexy	Improved	Improved	N/A
9.0 M	82.6	82.6	Palate asymmetry	H/A, sensory	N/A	Tonsils untouched	Improved	Improved	Increased
17.1 M	3.2	3.2	Normal	H/A	Presyrinx	Dural splitting	Improved	No change	Improved
4.8 M	29.0	29.0	Normal	H/A, dysphagia	Presyrinx	Dural splitting	Improved	Improved	Improved
12.5 F	23.1	23.1	Normal	None	C3-T9	Dural splitting	Improved	No change	Resolved
13.2 M	41.8	41.8	Normal	H/A	N/A	Dural splitting	Improved	Improved	N/A

Abbreviations: H/A, headache; N/A, not available.
[a] Age measured in years.
[b] Follow-up length measured in months.
[c] Patient did not have surgery (age at presentation).
[d] Incidental finding during evaluation for seizures.

finding was not significant (*P* = .43) (see **Table 2**). Two patients in the dural splitting cohort experienced minimal improvement postoperatively and required positive airway pressure as of most recent follow-up. In total, 3 patients underwent repeat surgery. Two (67%) patients in the duraplasty group exhibited symptomatic improvement but underwent repeat duraplasty (both tonisllopexy), 1 for an expansile syrinx and the other for a pseudomeningocele. One (25%) patient in the dural splitting group went on to receive duraplasty 9 months later for persistent symptoms and tonsillar herniation. All 3 of the patients who underwent repeat surgery showed improvement in sleep apnea at last follow-up. Postoperative complications included nausea/vomiting (n = 2), somnolence (n = 1, duraplasty), and significant neck pain with slow ambulation (n = 1, dural splitting). Median length of hospital stay was 4.0 (range 3.0–71.0) days for duraplasty and 3.5 (range 2.0–5.0) days for dural splitting. Median postoperative ICU length was 1.0 (range 1.0–25.0) day for duraplasty and 1.0 day (for all patients) for dural splitting. One patient with duraplasty had significant postoperative complications that required tracheostomy and longer-term care in the pediatric rehabilitation center.

Evaluation of Cerebrospinal Fluid Flow

CSF flow at the foramen magnum was evaluated in all 8 patients at the time of CM-1 diagnosis. All patients (100%) exhibited abnormal CSF flow during the initial imaging study. One patient in the duraplasty group exhibited mild improvement in CSF flow compared with initial MRI. A higher proportion of dural splitting patients exhibited improved CSF flow on follow-up imaging (100% of patients who underwent repeat studies). A change in CSF flow analysis was not used as a surgical indication in this series of patients.

CLINICAL RESULTS IN THE LITERATURE

Pediatric patients with CM-1 can present with a diverse spectrum of symptoms secondary to PFD. Tonsillar herniation can result in compression of the afferent, efferent, and/or central respiratory control pathways within the brainstem and manifest clinically in acute respiratory failure, central and obstructive apnea, and/or hypopnea. The association between Chiari malformation with tonsillar herniation and sleep apnea has been previously described in several series, although these have been limited mostly to adult populations.[6–10] Botelho and colleagues[33] reported an incidence of sleep apnea (defined as apnea-hypopnea index >5) of 44% and 60% in 23 patients with

CM-1 with and without syringomyelia, respectively (compared with 12% in the control group, n = 12). The same group previously reported that 72% of 11 patients with CM-1 presented with (predominately central) sleep apnea.[34] Another series by Gagnadoux and colleagues[27] illustrated sleep apnea (apnea-hypopnea index >10) in 75% of 16 adult patients with CM-1. Central apneic events ranged from 17% to 48% in both cases. A more recent report of 46 patients (20 children and adults) identified sleep apnea in 70% of CM-1 patients composed mainly of children.[14] Relatively few reports describe the frequency, severity, and underlying pathophysiology of respiratory disturbances in CM-1, particularly in the pediatric population.

Without generally accepted criteria for selecting patients with CM-1 for surgical treatment, coupled with the diverse constellation of symptoms associated with CM-1, the decision for and technique of surgery can be somewhat provisional. Although surgical decompression serves as the preferred treatment of sleep apnea in patients with Chiari malformation, the effect of surgery differs among patients, and respiratory failure can become a complication of treatment.[6,8,9,21–26] Similarly, there is a dearth of literature describing and comparing different approaches to and the nuances of PFD for CM-1 and their respective outcomes, particularly with respect to concurrent sleep apnea.

In this study of a cohort of 8 pediatric patients diagnosed with concurrent CM-1 and sleep apnea, 1 patient was treated conservatively and 7 patients underwent posterior fossa decompression. Of these 7 surgical patients, 3 were treated with duraplasty and 4 were treated with a dural splitting technique. Surgical intervention was associated with improvement of symptoms and radiographic evidence of tonsillar ectopia and syringomyelia. Overall, surgery improved sleep apnea in 62.5% of patients (100% of the duraplasty group and 50% of the dural splitting group). In reference to surgical technique, there was no statistically significant difference in resolution of sleep apnea between duraplasty and dural splitting techniques (*P* = .43), although this was likely secondary to the low study power of 7 surgical patients. Duraplasty and dural splitting were both associated with a notable reduction in tonsillar herniation of 58% and 24%, respectively (duraplasty excluding tonsillectomy was associated with a mean reduction of 37%).

These findings are consistent with the prevailing literature comparing more versus less invasive modes of Chiari decompression. In recent years, several neurosurgical series have compared extradural PFD to duraplasty with mixed evidence to suggest any significant difference in symptomatic outcome.[35–38] Limonadi and Selden[35] reported the relative safety, good early clinical results, and significantly reduced resource use for dural splitting in 24 pediatric patients with CM-1. Navarro and colleagues[36] advocated for a tailored posterior fossa craniectomy with dural scoring as the initial surgical procedure in children with CM-1 with or without syrinx because this minimized postoperative complications associated with dural opening and offered comparable rates of success in 96 patients (72% for PFD with bony decompression and dural scoring vs 68% for duraplasty). Although recent series have described patients with or without syringomyelia, symptoms considered were largely confined to headache, sensorimotor disturbance, dysphagia, and nausea/vomiting and did not include patients with sleep apnea.

Lee and colleagues[39] provided a balanced treatment comparison focusing on long-term clinical outcome and radiographic syrinx improvement and proposed that extradural decompression for CM-1 leads to comparable clinical and radiographic improvement compared with traditional PFD with duraplasty (PFDD) but offers decreased postoperative morbidity. The investigators recommended more invasive PFDD as first-line treatment of more severe patients with rapidly progressive symptoms or severe neurologic deficits. Because PFD with dural augmentation has become the traditional procedure of choice in most centers, there has been increasing advocacy for the use of a less invasive extradural decompression[39–43] secondary to shorter lengths of operation and hospital admission as well as reduced pain, morbidity, and CSF-related complications.[35–37,40,42,44–46] The authors' institutional experience echoes the prospect that dural splitting portends quicker and easier recovery for pediatric patients. Despite the advantage of avoiding a more invasive procedure, some recent reports have associated extradural decompression with higher rates of surgical revision for patients with persistent underlying malformations.[36,40,46–49] Controversy also persists with regards to treating syringomyelia.[40,50]

Insofar as specific decision criteria for identifying suitable patients with CM-1 for decompression remains contentious, so too does surgical technique. That bony decompression alone rarely suffices in restoring CSF circulation at the cervico-occipital junction[51–53] may be not only a byproduct of the thickened dura in CM-1[54] but also because dura in the posterior fossa cannot reliably expand when left wholly intact.[55] Recent series supporting intradural techniques, such as CSF shunting of the fourth ventricle, ablation, or

retraction of the cerebellar tonsils, have tempered decent results with potentially unnecessary risks of meningocele, meningitis, and delayed wound healing.[55–58] Complications secondary to CSF leaks have been reported in approximately 16% of cases with dural grafts without arachnoid opening.[59] Earlier reports of duraplasty with arachnoid opening have been associated with aseptic meningitis and CSF leaks in 36% and 32% of surgical patients, respectively.[60]

The original account of an extradural approach to removing the outer dural layer by Isu and colleagues[61] in 1993 included 7 patients, 6 of whom improved with surgical management and experienced no postoperative complications. A more recent report of dural splitting showed similar improvement in symptoms in 11 patients with CM-1 (5 with syringomyelia), including headaches, cervicalgias, dizziness, and parasthesias, with only 1 postoperative complication manifesting as a minor superficial wound infection.[55] Although investigators have proposed that dural splitting often fails to completely resolve symptoms associated with more severe degrees of tonsillar herniation, such as below the level of C2, dural splitting has precluded the need for repeat surgery.[55,56,62] In pediatric patients, dural splitting has wielded positive results.[35,63,64] Despite these positive results, the authors' findings suggest that revision surgery is certainly a risk with duraplasty (67% of patients) and, to a lesser extent, dural splitting (25%); so caution should be taken when choosing appropriate patients for these techniques.

To the authors' knowledge, there are no other published reports directly comparing duraplasty and dural splitting with long-term outcomes of patients with concurrent sleep apnea and CM-1. Literature describing symptomatic control of sleep apnea in patients with CM-1 remains sparse. Previous reports based on isolated cases have demonstrated improvement of central sleep apnea after surgical correction.[6,65,66] Gagnadoux and colleagues[27] reported a series of 12 patients with CM-1 whose average apnea-hypopnea index declined from 56.5 to 37.2 and central apnea index from 14.9 to 1.3 after surgical decompression. Botelho and colleagues[67] reported clinically beneficial improvement in polysomnographic values (>50% decrease) in 47% of 17 patients with sleep apnea. The investigators proposed that surgery was associated with a significant improvement in the mean number of respiratory events, obstructive events, central events, apnea-hypopnea index, and central apnea index, with a more pronounced effected in patients with central sleep apnea.

The longitudinal nature of follow-up and multidisciplinary evaluation and care lend credence to the comparison of PFD technique in children with sleep apnea as part of a CM-1 diagnosis. Comprehensive neurologic and radiographic examinations were instrumental in confirming prospective diagnoses of CM-1 and concurrent syringomyelia as well as identifying appropriate surgical candidates.

Going forward, longitudinal follow-up studies with special emphasis on patients with either neurologic deficits or severe symptoms, such as sleep apnea, despite widespread acceptance of decompression in these patients, will help to further elucidate the natural history of CM-1 and more appropriately gauge the risk-benefit tradeoff of a growing spectrum of surgical interventions. PFD technique and resolution of sleep apnea in CM-1 should be explored with more patients. Further study over longer time horizons meant to capture all cases of clinical and/or radiographic deterioration may further be able to refine diagnostic criteria, predict symptomatic progression, and accordingly match appropriate surgical and nonsurgical therapeutic modalities to patient functioning.

SUMMARY

Duraplasty and dural splitting are associated with radiographic and symptomatic improvement in pediatric patients with concurrent sleep-related breathing disorders and CM-1. Central sleep apnea represents an indication for surgical decompression in these patients.

SUPPLEMENTARY DATA

Supplementary data related to this article can be found online at http://dx.doi.org/10.1016/j.nec.2015.06.009.

REFERENCES

1. Dhamija R, Wetjen NM, Slocumb NL, et al. The role of nocturnal polysomnography in assessing children with Chiari type I malformation. Clin Neurol Neurosurg 2013;115(9):1837–41.
2. Speer MC, George TM, Enterline DS, et al. A genetic hypothesis for Chiari I malformation with or without syringomyelia. Neurosurg Focus 2000;8(3):E12.
3. Strahle J, Muraszko KM, Kapurch J, et al. Chiari malformation Type I and syrinx in children undergoing magnetic resonance imaging. J Neurosurg Pediatr 2011;8(2):205–13.
4. Steinbok P. Clinical features of Chiari I malformations. Childs Nerv Syst 2004;20(5):329–31.
5. Benglis D Jr, Covington D, Bhatia R, et al. Outcomes in pediatric patients with Chiari malformation Type I followed up without surgery. J Neurosurg Pediatr 2011;7(4):375–9.
6. Zolty P, Sanders MH, Pollack IF. Chiari malformation and sleep-disordered breathing: a review of diagnostic and management issues. Sleep 2000;23(5):637–43.
7. Alvarez D, Requena I, Arias M, et al. Acute respiratory failure as the first sign of Arnold-Chiari malformation associated with syringomyelia. Eur Respir J 1995;8(4):661–3.
8. Shiihara T, Shimizu Y, Mitsui T, et al. Isolated sleep apnea due to Chiari type I malformation and syringomyelia. Pediatr Neurol 1995;13(3):266–7.
9. Rabec C, Laurent G, Baudouin N, et al. Central sleep apnoea in Arnold-Chiari malformation: evidence of pathophysiological heterogeneity. Eur Respir J 1998;12(6):1482–5.
10. Yglesias A, Narbona J, Vanaclocha V, et al. Chiari type I malformation, glossopharyngeal neuralgia and central sleep apnoea in a child. Dev Med Child Neurol 1996;38(12):1126–30.
11. Ali NJ, Pitson DJ, Stradling JR. Snoring, sleep disturbance, and behaviour in 4-5 year olds. Arch Dis Child 1993;68(3):360–6.
12. Montgomery-Downs HE, O'Brien LM, Gulliver TE, et al. Polysomnographic characteristics in normal preschool and early school-aged children. Pediatrics 2006;117(3):741–53.
13. Traeger N, Schultz B, Pollock AN, et al. Polysomnographic values in children 2-9 years old: additional data and review of the literature. Pediatr Pulmonol 2005;40(1):22–30.
14. Dauvilliers Y, Stal V, Abril B, et al. Chiari malformation and sleep related breathing disorders. J Neurol Neurosurg Psychiatry 2007;78(12):1344–8.
15. Aarts LA, Willemsen MA, Vandenbussche NL, et al. Nocturnal apnea in Chiari type I malformation. Eur J Pediatr 2011;170(10):1349–52.
16. Gosalakkal JA. Sleep-disordered breathing in Chiari malformation type 1. Pediatr Neurol 2008;39(3):207–8.
17. Murray C, Seton C, Prelog K, et al. Arnold Chiari type 1 malformation presenting with sleep disordered breathing in well children. Arch Dis Child 2006;91(4):342–3.
18. Van den Broek MJ, Arbues AS, Chalard F, et al. Chiari type I malformation causing central apnoeas in a 4-month-old boy. Eur J Paediatr Neurol 2009;13(5):463–5.
19. Wealthall SR, Whittaker GE, Greenwood N. The relationship of apnoea and stridor in spina bifida to other unexplained infant deaths. Dev Med Child Neurol 1974;16(6 Suppl 32):107–16.
20. Tubbs RS, Lyerly MJ, Loukas M, et al. The pediatric Chiari I malformation: a review. Childs Nerv Syst 2007;23(11):1239–50.
21. Paul KS, Lye RH, Strang FA, et al. Arnold-Chiari malformation. Review of 71 cases. J Neurosurg 1983;58(2):183–7.

22. Omer S, al-Kawi MZ, Bohlega S, et al. Respiratory arrest: a complication of Arnold-Chiari malformation in adults. Eur Neurol 1996;36(1):36–8.

23. Tsara V, Serasli E, Kimiskidis V, et al. Acute respiratory failure and sleep-disordered breathing in Arnold-Chiari malformation. Clin Neurol Neurosurg 2005;107(6):521–4.

24. Doherty MJ, Spence DP, Young C, et al. Obstructive sleep apnoea with Arnold-Chiari malformation. Thorax 1995;50(6):690–1 [discussion: 696–7].

25. Bokinsky GE, Hudson LD, Weil JV. Impaired peripheral chemosensitivity and acute respiratory failure in Arnold-Chiari malformation and syringomyelia. N Engl J Med 1973;288(18):947–8.

26. Ely EW, McCall WV, Haponik EF. Multifactorial obstructive sleep apnea in a patient with Chiari malformation. J Neurol Sci 1994;126(2):232–6.

27. Gagnadoux F, Meslier N, Svab I, et al. Sleep-disordered breathing in patients with Chiari malformation: improvement after surgery. Neurology 2006;66(1):136–8.

28. Wu YW, Chin CT, Chan KM, et al. Pediatric Chiari I malformations: do clinical and radiologic features correlate? Neurology 1999;53(6):1271–6.

29. Aboulezz AO, Sartor K, Geyer CA, et al. Position of cerebellar tonsils in the normal population and in patients with Chiari malformation: a quantitative approach with MR imaging. J Comput Assist Tomogr 1985;9(6):1033–6.

30. Aitken LA, Lindan CE, Sidney S, et al. Chiari type I malformation in a pediatric population. Pediatr Neurol 2009;40(6):449–54.

31. Barkovich AJ, Wippold FJ, Sherman JL, et al. Significance of cerebellar tonsillar position on MR. AJNR Am J Neuroradiol 1986;7(5):795–9.

32. Novegno F, Caldarelli M, Massa A, et al. The natural history of the Chiari Type I anomaly. J Neurosurg Pediatr 2008;2(3):179–87.

33. Botelho RV, Bittencourt LR, Rotta JM, et al. A prospective controlled study of sleep respiratory events in patients with craniovertebral junction malformation. J Neurosurg 2003;99(6):1004–9.

34. Botelho RV, Bittencourt LR, Rotta JM, et al. Polysomnographic respiratory findings in patients with Arnold-Chiari type I malformation and basilar invagination, with or without syringomyelia: preliminary report of a series of cases. Neurosurg Rev 2000;23(3):151–5.

35. Limonadi FM, Selden NR. Dura-splitting decompression of the craniocervical junction: reduced operative time, hospital stay, and cost with equivalent early outcome. J Neurosurg 2004;101(2 Suppl):184–8.

36. Navarro R, Olavarria G, Seshadri R, et al. Surgical results of posterior fossa decompression for patients with Chiari I malformation. Childs Nerv Syst 2004;20(5):349–56.

37. Munshi I, Frim D, Stine-Reyes R, et al. Effects of posterior fossa decompression with and without duraplasty on Chiari malformation-associated hydromyelia. Neurosurgery 2000;46(6):1384–9 [discussion: 1389–90].

38. McGirt MJ, Attenello FJ, Atiba A, et al. Symptom recurrence after suboccipital decompression for pediatric Chiari I malformation: analysis of 256 consecutive cases. Childs Nerv Syst 2008;24(11):1333–9.

39. Lee A, Yarbrough CK, Greenberg JK, et al. Comparison of posterior fossa decompression with or without duraplasty in children with Type I Chiari malformation. Childs Nerv Syst 2014;30(8):1419–24.

40. Durham SR, Fjeld-Olenec K. Comparison of posterior fossa decompression with and without duraplasty for the surgical treatment of Chiari malformation Type I in pediatric patients: a meta-analysis. J Neurosurg Pediatr 2008;2(1):42–9.

41. Alzate JC, Kothbauer KF, Jallo GI, et al. Treatment of Chiari I malformation in patients with and without syringomyelia: a consecutive series of 66 cases. Neurosurg Focus 2001;11(1):E3.

42. Galarza M, Sood S, Ham S. Relevance of surgical strategies for the management of pediatric Chiari type I malformation. Childs Nerv Syst 2007;23(6):691–6.

43. Park JK, Gleason PL, Madsen JR, et al. Presentation and management of Chiari I malformation in children. Pediatr Neurosurg 1997;26(4):190–6.

44. Caldarelli M, Novegno F, Vassimi L, et al. The role of limited posterior fossa craniectomy in the surgical treatment of Chiari malformation Type I: experience with a pediatric series. J Neurosurg 2007;106(3 Suppl):187–95.

45. Erdogan E, Cansever T, Secer HI, et al. The evaluation of surgical treatment options in the Chiari Malformation Type I. Turk Neurosurg 2010;20(3):303–13.

46. Ramirez LF, Thisted R. Using a national health care data base to determine surgical complications in community hospitals: lumbar discectomy as an example. Neurosurgery 1989;25(2):218–25.

47. Yeh DD, Koch B, Crone KR. Intraoperative ultrasonography used to determine the extent of surgery necessary during posterior fossa decompression in children with Chiari malformation type I. J Neurosurg 2006;105(1 Suppl):26–32.

48. Aliaga L, Hekman KE, Yassari R, et al. A novel scoring system for assessing Chiari malformation type I treatment outcomes. Neurosurgery 2012;70(3):656–64 [discussion: 664–5].

49. Yarbrough CK, Greenberg JK, Smyth MD, et al. External validation of the Chicago Chiari Outcome Scale. J Neurosurg Pediatr 2014;13(6):679–84.

50. Rocque BG, George TM, Kestle J, et al. Treatment practices for Chiari malformation type I with syringomyelia: results of a survey of the American Society of

Pediatric Neurosurgeons. J Neurosurg Pediatr 2011; 8(5):430–7.

51. Balagura S, Kuo DC. Spontaneous retraction of cerebellar tonsils after surgery for Arnold-Chiari malformation and posterior fossa cyst. Surg Neurol 1988;29(2):137–40.

52. Milhorat TH, Bolognese PA. Tailored operative technique for Chiari type I malformation using intraoperative color Doppler ultrasonography. Neurosurgery 2003;53(4):899–905 [discussion: 905–6].

53. Raftopoulos C, Sanchez A, Matos C, et al. Hydrosyringomyelia-Chiari I complex. Prospective evaluation of a modified foramen magnum decompression procedure: preliminary results. Surg Neurol 1993;39(2):163–9.

54. Nakamura N, Iwasaki Y, Hida K, et al. Dural band pathology in syringomyelia with Chiari type I malformation. Neuropathology 2000;20(1):38–43.

55. Chauvet D, Carpentier A, George B. Dura splitting decompression in Chiari type 1 malformation: clinical experience and radiological findings. Neurosurg Rev 2009;32(4):465–70.

56. Batzdorf U. Chiari I malformation with syringomyelia. Evaluation of surgical therapy by magnetic resonance imaging. J Neurosurg 1988;68(5):726–30.

57. Belen D, Er U, Gurses L, et al. Delayed pseudomyelomeningocele: a rare complication after foramen magnum decompression for Chiari malformation. Surg Neurol 2009;71(3):357–61 [discussion: 361].

58. Dones J, De Jesus O, Colen CB, et al. Clinical outcomes in patients with Chiari I malformation: a review of 27 cases. Surg Neurol 2003;60(2):142–7 [discussion: 147–8].

59. Sindou M, Chavez-Machuca J, Hashish H. Craniocervical decompression for Chiari type I-malformation, adding extreme lateral foramen magnum opening and expansile duroplasty with arachnoid preservation. Technique and long-term functional results in 44 consecutive adult cases – comparison with literature data. Acta Neurochir (Wien) 2002; 144(10):1005–19.

60. Klekamp J, Batzdorf U, Samii M, et al. The surgical treatment of Chiari I malformation. Acta Neurochir (Wien) 1996;138(7):788–801.

61. Isu T, Sasaki H, Takamura H, et al. Foramen magnum decompression with removal of the outer layer of the dura as treatment for syringomyelia occurring with Chiari I malformation. Neurosurgery 1993;33(5): 845–9 [discussion: 849–50].

62. Badie B, Mendoza D, Batzdorf U. Posterior fossa volume and response to suboccipital decompression in patients with Chiari I malformation. Neurosurgery 1995;37(2):214–8.

63. Genitori L, Peretta P, Nurisso C, et al. Chiari type I anomalies in children and adolescents: minimally invasive management in a series of 53 cases. Childs Nerv Syst 2000;16(10–11):707–18.

64. Hida K, Iwasaki Y, Koyanagi I, et al. Surgical indication and results of foramen magnum decompression versus syringosubarachnoid shunting for syringomyelia associated with Chiari I malformation. Neurosurgery 1995;37(4):673–8 [discussion: 678–9].

65. Lam B, Ryan CF. Arnold-Chiari malformation presenting as sleep apnea syndrome. Sleep Med 2000;1(2):139–44.

66. Botelho RV, Bittencourt LR, Rotta JM, et al. Adult Chiari malformation and sleep apnoea. Neurosurg Rev 2005;28(3):169–76.

67. Botelho RV, Bittencourt LR, Rotta JM, et al. The effects of posterior fossa decompressive surgery in adult patients with Chiari malformation and sleep apnea. J Neurosurg 2010;112(4):800–7.

Complex Chiari Malformations in Children: Diagnosis and Management

Douglas L. Brockmeyer, MD*, Heather S. Spader, MD

KEYWORDS

- Complex Chiari • Basilar invagination • Clivocervical angle • Retroflexed odontoid

KEY POINTS

- Complex Chiari malformations may be a distinct category from other Chiari malformations.
- These patients are at increased risk for occipitocervical fusions after Chiari decompression or may need upfront decompression and fusion procedures.
- The decision-making algorithm for these patients needs to be modified to account for different outcomes for these patients. This algorithm includes clinical symptoms, extent of Chiari, evaluation of clival-cervical angle, retroflexed odontoid, and basilar invagination.

DEFINITION OF COMPLEX CHIARI MALFORMATION

Chiari malformations were originally classified by Chiari in 1896 into three categories based on anatomic description[1]:

- Chiari 1: Cerebellar tonsil and lower part of the medulla below the foramen magnum without displacement of the fourth ventricle.
- Chiari 2: Caudal migration of the lower part of the cerebellum associated with downward displacement of the fourth ventricle, which appears lengthened; foramina opens into the spinal subarachnoid space; associated with spina bifida.
- Chiari 3: Cerebellum and medulla displaced into the cervical spinal canal associated with an occipital meningocele.

Later, a fourth type was added that describes an incomplete or underdeveloped cerebellum.

These categories were clinically useful for almost 100 years; however, as neurosurgeons began studying outcome data for surgical decompression of Chiari 1 malformations (C1M), it became apparent that there was a subcategory of patients in whom the condition was more complex; these patients required more frequent surgical intervention than the others. Initial examination of this group by Grabb and colleagues[2] in 1999 showed that odontoid retroflexion, manifested by a pBC2 distance (maximum perpendicular distance to the basion-inferoposterior point of the C2 body) greater than 9 mm, defined a patient group that frequently required craniocervical fusion procedures. Further experience with this patient population led to the observation that a subcategory of patients with Chiari malformation had caudal descent of the brainstem and tonsillar ectopia. Therefore, a new category, the Chiari 1.5 malformation (C1.5M), was proposed; it was defined as the presence of obex herniation below the foramen magnum as seen on MRI.[3]

With a growing awareness of the complex nature of disease in some Chiari patients, Bollo and colleagues[4] comprehensively analyzed their experience with patients that manifested a constellation of craniospinal radiographic findings

Division of Pediatric Neurosurgery, Primary Children's Hospital, University of Utah, 100 Mario Capecchi Drive, Salt Lake City, UT 84113, USA
* Corresponding author.
E-mail address: Douglas.Brockmeyer@hsc.utah.edu

Neurosurg Clin N Am 26 (2015) 555–560
http://dx.doi.org/10.1016/j.nec.2015.06.002
1042-3680/15/$ – see front matter © 2015 Elsevier Inc. All rights reserved.

aside from just tonsillar herniation. These findings included

- Brainstem herniation through the foramen magnum (C1.5M)
- Medullary kink
- Retroflexed odontoid
- Abnormal clival-cervical angle (CXA)
- Occipitalization of the atlas
- Basilar invagination (BI)
- Syringomyelia
- Scoliosis

The authors analyzed a group of patients with the previously mentioned radiographic findings and found that the presence of a C1.5M, a CXA less than 125°, and BI placed a patient at a higher risk for requiring a craniocervical fusion than those with a typical C1M. They proposed a new category of Chiari malformation, known as complex Chiari malformation (CCM), that encompasses these radiographic findings, all or in part. Further detail about these measurements is illustrated in **Fig. 1**. Although there are several previous case series in the literature describing the management of complex-type Chiari patients,[5–10] Bollo and colleagues[4] were the first to analyze a large group of patients with CCM and define factors that place patients at a higher risk for craniocervical fusion. Here, we describe the diagnostic criteria for CCM and outline the decision-making process for the optimal treatment of this patient population.

PATIENT SELECTION
Clinical Findings

In general, the clinical presentation of patients with CCM is not much different from that of typical C1M

patients. They tend to present with lifestyle-limiting headaches, often in the suboccipital region. Paresthesias or bulbomyelopathic symptoms, such sleep apnea, snoring, dysphagia, or ataxia, are often found. Patients younger than 4 years of age often present with symptoms consistent with oral-motor apraxia (eg, poor feeding, delayed speech) and/or apnea.[4,11]

Radiographic Findings

To identify a CCM, the initial craniospinal MRI must be evaluated for

- Chiari1.5M
- Odontoid retroflexion, measured by pBC2 (**Fig. 2**)
- CXA
- BI
- Assimilation of the atlas
- Medullary kinking

Other findings may include hydrocephalus, associated brain abnormalities, scoliosis, and syringomyelia. Together, these radiographic elements identify a CCM and help the clinician make decisions about proceeding with surgery.

Clinical-Radiographic Integration

Step 1: surgical decision making
First, the surgeon must decide whether the patient's symptoms are severe enough to warrant surgery. A useful distinction is to ask the patient whether the problem is truly lifestyle limiting. For children, this means the symptoms keep them home from school, prevent them from doing something they normally enjoy (such as playing with friends), or cause them to quit early from their

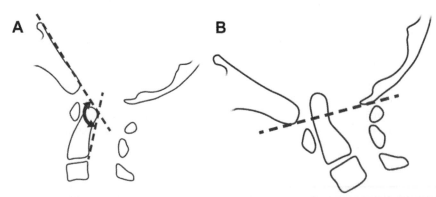

Fig. 1. Illustration of clival-cervical angle. This is the angle (*double arrow*) derived from a line drawn from the inferior two-thirds of the clivus and a second line drawn from the posterior-inferior C2 body to the superior-posterior aspect of the odontoid (*A*). Basilar invagination is seen when the odontoid process of C2 is above the foramen magnum. McRae's line is the line joining the basion and opisthion. The dens should normally be 5 mm below this line (*B*).

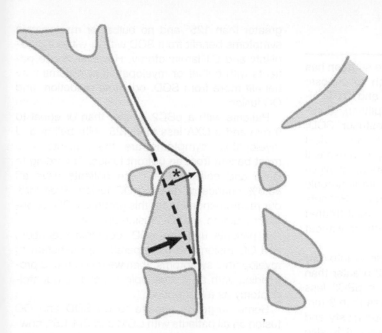

Fig. 2. Illustration of pBC2 line. A line is drawn from the inferior portion of the clivus to the posterior-inferior aspect of the C2 vertebral body (*arrow*). The pBC2 distance (*double arrow*) is from that line to the posterior superior aspect of the odontoid process (*asterisk*) of C2.

normal activities. If the Chiari malformation is an incidental finding or discovered during the work-up for scoliosis, however, the surgeon must decide whether the radiographic findings are concerning enough that a procedure is indicated. Such is frequently the case when syringomyelia is found in conjunction with scoliosis. In the authors' opinion, all patients with moderate to large syrinxes, with or without scoliosis, should be offered surgery. The long-term outlook for patients with significant syringomyelia is unfavorable enough that a decompressive Chiari surgery is a prudent option.[12,13] Patients with small syrinxes and mild scoliosis may be safely monitored with serial scanning. There are obviously no hard-and-fast rules in this decision-making process. Clinical judgment must be exercised for each patient, but by developing general evidence-based treatment principles in one's mind, the discussion process with the patient's family is easier, and appropriate solutions may be offered for each child.

Step 2: radiologic evaluation
The radiographic parameters listed previously must be sequentially evaluated and stratified into risk categories that help make surgical decisions. Typically in a patient with a CCM, C1.5M with medullary kinking is present. BI is also seen frequently, but it is not always present. The existence of BI, according to Bollo and colleagues,[4] places the patient in a higher-risk category for craniocervical fusion, but it is not a primary reason to offer surgery. Axis assimilation is also often noted,

but independently is also not a primary indication for craniocervical fusion.

After these findings are considered, the degree of odontoid retroflexion (pBC2) and CXA are evaluated. Together, they are the primary radiographic factors that drive decisions in the CCM patient. Odontoid retroflexion has been shown to be associated with the need for craniocervical fusion,[2] but its absolute value seems to make little difference in patient presentation, except in extreme cases. The complex interplay between odontoid retroflexion and craniocervical kyphosis is the critical component. Bollo and colleagues[4] showed that the combination of a CXA of less than 125° (measured by the method in their study) or less than 135° (measured by the method described by Grabb and colleagues[2]) and a retroflexed odontoid is the primary driver of progressive craniocervical kyphosis and is predictive of the need for craniocervical fusion.[2,4] This certainly is the case for patients with CCM in whom the initial standard posterior suboccipital decompression (SOD) procedure fails, given that the posterior craniocervical musculoligamentous tension band has been released. Releasing the posterior tension band allows progressive craniocervical settling and kyphosis to occur. As a result, some patients never make a full recovery after their initial procedure. They complain of headache, neck pain, and fatigue. Sometimes bulbar findings occur or worsen compared with their baseline state. Ultimately, craniocervical stabilization with odontoid reduction is required to restore craniocervical alignment and reduce anterior brainstem compression.

OPERATIVE INTERVENTION
Patient-Treatment Algorithm

Faced with a patient with a CCM, the surgeon has a variety of procedures from which to choose: standard suboccipital craniectomy and C1 laminectomy (with or without dural splitting, duraplasty, and tonsillar shrinking); posterior SOD, duraplasty, odontoid reduction, occipitocervical (OC) fusion; or tansoral or endoscopic transnasal odontoid resection. The patient-treatment algorithm in **Fig. 3** integrates the clinicoradiographic findings with the surgical procedures. Patients who present with a simple CM1 are best treated with SOD and C1 laminectomy with or without duraplasty.

Patients with a CCM can be divided into two initial categories: those with a pBC2 greater than or equal to 9 mm and those with a pBC2 less than 9 mm. Patients with a pBC2 less than 9 mm benefit from SOD with or without duraplasty and a C1 laminectomy. For these patients, it is also important to document the CXA. Although this angle does not necessarily help with the initial surgical decision, it does inform the patient and surgeon about possible future OC fusion risk. Patients with a CXA greater than or equal to 125° have a 1.7% future fusion risk, whereas those with a CXA less than 125° have a 13% future fusion risk.[4]

For those patients with a pBC2 greater than or equal to 9 mm, the CXA is the next important factor in making surgical decisions. Patients with a CXA greater than 125° and no bulbar or myelopathic symptoms benefit from SOD with or without duraplasty and C1 laminectomy. However, those patients with bulbar or myelopathic symptoms may benefit more from SOD, odontoid reduction, and OC fusion.

Patients with a pBC2 greater than or equal to 9 mm and a CXA less than 125° with bulbar and myelopathic symptoms are the patients who most benefit from an upfront fusion. According to Bollo and colleagues,[4] these patients have an 83.3% chance of needing OC fusion. Therefore, our recommendation for this group is SOD, odontoid reduction, and OC fusion upfront.

If patients undergo SOD, odontoid reduction, and OC fusion and have persisting brainstem or myelopathic symptoms, then we recommend proceeding with an endoscopic endonasal odontoidectomy as a last option.

Some surgeons choose to do SOD and OC fusion on all patients with CCM and CM 1.5[6]; however, we believe that it may be more beneficial to stratify the patients in a stepwise fashion according to clinical and radiographic criteria and have a conversation with the family about the overall lifetime risk of OC fusion.[4]

Operative Procedures

A discussion of the merits of each operative procedure for CCM is beyond the scope of this article; however, a few brief comments are called for

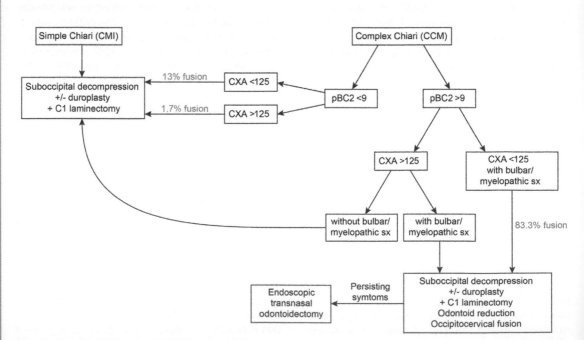

Fig. 3. Complex Chiari management algorithm.

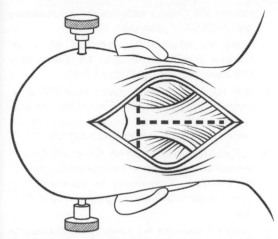

Fig. 4. Illustration of T-shaped incision in the fascia facilitating an easier closure.

when operative management for a CCM is required.

1. SOD, C1 laminectomy, tonsillar shrinking, and duraplasty
   a. The senior author prefers a T-shaped opening in the suboccipital musculature (**Fig. 4**). This makes for a better, tighter closure after the procedure is done.
   b. Too much occipital bone removal is a mistake. The craniectomy should typically be limited to about 3 cm wide and 3 cm high. This amount of bone removal allows adequate room for intradural exploration while keeping enough bone laterally so that if a subsequent OC fusion is required, the instrumentation can be placed easily. Approximately 3 cm of the posterior C1 lamina should be removed as well.

   c. Be sure of adequate bony removal around the foramen magnum. This is, after all, a skull-base surgery.
   d. Needless to say, great care must be used when dissecting free and shrinking the tonsils using electrocautery. The lateral portion of the tonsils, near the 11th nerve, should be freed up and shrunk as well to allow for better circumferential flow of cerebrospinal fluid postoperatively.
   e. The outlet to the fourth ventricle must be explored, and any obstruction, scarring, or banding must be opened.
   f. The less blood lost intradurally the better. Reducing blood loss is believed to reduce the incidence of postoperative chemical meningitis.
   g. The duraplasty must be watertight.

2. SOD, odontoid reduction, and craniocervical fusion (**Fig. 5**)
   a. The procedure proceeds as described previously.
   b. C2 pars screws are placed under fluoroscopic guidance to anchor the OC construct.
   c. OC instrumentation is cut and shaped to fit the OC contour.
   d. The occipital end of the construct is fixed.
   e. Manual intraoperative reduction is performed, with gentle distraction and extension of the head.
   f. The cervical portion of the construct is locked into place.
   g. Posterior rib autografts are harvested and contoured to fit between C2 and the occiput.
   h. Fusion adjuncts are used at the discretion of the surgeon. Recombinant human bone morphogenetic protein is not routinely

Fig. 5. Illustration of SOD, odontoid reduction, craniocervical fusion. Gray, occipitocervical fusion plates and rods; blue, C2 pars screws; pink, occipital screws.

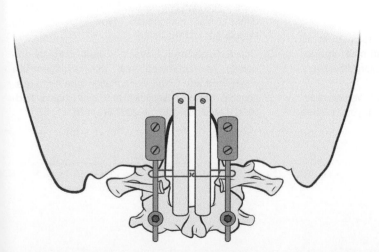

used, and if it is, only in small amounts at bone contact points.
3. Transnasal endoscopic odontoid resection
   a. It is important to enlist the assistance of an experienced otolaryngologic surgeon to assist in the approach, odontoid resection, and closure of the wound. An otolaryngologic surgeon is usually much more facile with intranasal endoscopic visualization than the typical neurosurgeon.
   b. Once a surgical corridor is established, the drilling out of C1 and the odontoid is fairly straightforward. Typically, only bony removal of the odontoid is necessary.
   c. The nasal mucosa is closed per the otolaryngologic surgeon. The postoperative management and hospital course of a patient is similar to a typical tonsillectomy and adenoidectomy case.

SUMMARY

The constellation of signs and symptoms comprising the CCM include brainstem herniation through the foramen magnum, medullary kinking, retroflexed odontoid, abnormal CXA, occipitalization of the atlas, BI, and syringomyelia. Affected patients can also, but not always, present with bulbar symptoms. Treatment of these patients is complicated by a higher risk for eventual fusion. Therefore, the pBC2 line and CXA are useful tools for making management decisions. Specifically, a patient with a pBC2 of greater than 9 mm and CXA less than 125° is most likely to need a Chiari decompression and cervical fusion. Patients with a normal pBC2 and CXA are likely to only need a Chiari decompression without fusion. Patients with values in between have to be evaluated individually based on their symptoms and risk for future fusion.

REFERENCES

1. Caetano de Barros M, Farias W, Ataide L, et al. Basilar impression and Arnold-Chiari malformation. A study of 66 cases. J Neurol Neurosurg Psychiatry 1968;31(6):596–605.
2. Grabb PA, Mapstone TB, Oakes WJ. Ventral brain stem compression in pediatric and young adult patients with Chiari I malformations. Neurosurgery 1999;44(3):520–7 [discussion: 527–8].
3. Tubbs RS, Iskandar BJ, Bartolucci AA, et al. A critical analysis of the Chiari 1.5 malformation. J Neurosurg 2004;101(2 Suppl):179–83.
4. Bollo RJ, Riva-Cambrin J, Brockmeyer MM, et al. Complex Chiari malformations in children: an analysis of preoperative risk factors for occipitocervical fusion. J Neurosurg Pediatr 2012;10(2):134–41.
5. Collignon FP, Cohen-Gadol AA, Krauss WE. Circumferential decompression of the foramen magnum for the treatment of syringomyelia associated with basilar invagination. Neurosurg Rev Jul 2004;27(3):168–72.
6. Fenoy AJ, Menezes AH, Fenoy KA. Craniocervical junction fusions in patients with hindbrain herniation and syringohydromyelia. J Neurosurg Spine 2008;9(1):1–9.
7. Goel A, Bhatjiwale M, Desai K. Basilar invagination: a study based on 190 surgically treated patients. J Neurosurg 1998;88(6):962–8.
8. Hwang SW, Heilman CB, Riesenburger RI, et al. C1-C2 arthrodesis after transoral odontoidectomy and suboccipital craniectomy for ventral brain stem compression in Chiari I patients. Eur Spine J 2008;17(9):1211–7.
9. Kim LJ, Rekate HL, Klopfenstein JD, et al. Treatment of basilar invagination associated with Chiari I malformations in the pediatric population: cervical reduction and posterior occipitocervical fusion. J Neurosurg 2004;101(2 Suppl):189–95.
10. Smith JS, Shaffrey CI, Abel MF, et al. Basilar invagination. Neurosurgery 2010;66(3 Suppl):39–47.
11. Albert GW, Menezes AH, Hansen DR, et al. Chiari malformation Type I in children younger than age 6 years: presentation and surgical outcome. J Neurosurg Pediatr 2010;5(6):554–61.
12. Tubbs RS, Beckman J, Naftel RP, et al. Institutional experience with 500 cases of surgically treated pediatric Chiari malformation Type I. J Neurosurg Pediatr 2011;7(3):248–56.
13. Ono A, Suetsuna F, Ueyama K, et al. Surgical outcomes in adult patients with syringomyelia associated with Chiari malformation type I: the relationship between scoliosis and neurological findings. J Neurosurg Spine 2007;6(3):216–21.

Craniovertebral Junction Instability in the Setting of Chiari I Malformation

Hannah E. Goldstein, MD*, Richard C.E. Anderson, MD

KEYWORDS

• Craniovertebral • Instability • Fusion • Complex Chiari • Basilar invagination

KEY POINTS

• Craniovertebral junction (CVJ) instability in the setting of Chiari I malformation (CMI) is a rare but clinically important finding, most often presenting as basilar invagination.
• The diagnosis of CVJ instability should be based on a combination of clinical and radiographic findings, including myelopathy, basilar invagination, ventral brainstem compression, and Chiari 1.5.
• In most cases, children found to have CVJ instability with basilar invagination should undergo attempts at preoperative or intraoperative reduction to minimize the need for anterior decompression.
• Most children with symptomatic CMI, even those presenting with signs of brainstem compression, do not have CVJ instability and will improve with a standard posterior fossa decompression alone.

INTRODUCTION

Almost all patients with symptomatic Chiari I malformation (CMI) can be successfully treated with standard posterior fossa decompression (**Fig. 1**). Large studies have shown that symptoms, including those associated with basilar invagination and syringomyelia, are likely to improve with decompression alone, with or without duraplasty.[1–4] However, a small subset of patients will have radiographic and clinical evidence of craniovertebral junction (CVJ) instability on initial presentation and will require stabilization (**Fig. 2**). Furthermore, some patients will either fail to improve after an initial decompression or may progressively worsen over time. Some of these patients will be subsequently diagnosed with CVJ instability and will also require stabilization (**Fig. 3**).

Brockmeyer[4] recently defined the complex Chiari malformation as "cerebellar tonsil herniation combined with one or more of the following radiographic findings: brainstem herniation through the foramen magnum (Chiari 1.5 malformation), medullary kink, retroflexed odontoid, abnormal clival-cervical angle, occipitalization of the atlas, basilar invagination, syringomyelia or scoliosis." The investigators further differentiated complex Chiari malformation patients from typical CMI patients as being more likely to require further surgical interventions beyond a standard suboccipital decompression, including odontoid resection and CVJ stabilization.[4]

This article will:

1. Define CVJ instability and indications for stabilization in the setting of CMI based on a

Disclosure: The authors report no conflict of interest concerning the materials or methods used in this study or the findings specified in this article.

Department of Neurosurgery, Morgan Stanley Children's Hospital of New York, The Neurologic Institute, Columbia University, 710 W. 168th Street, New York, NY 10032, USA

* Corresponding author. The Neurological Institute, Columbia University Medical Center, 710 West 168th Street, 4th Floor, New York, NY 10032.

E-mail address: heg2117@columbia.edu

Neurosurg Clin N Am 26 (2015) 561–569

http://dx.doi.org/10.1016/j.nec.2015.06.001

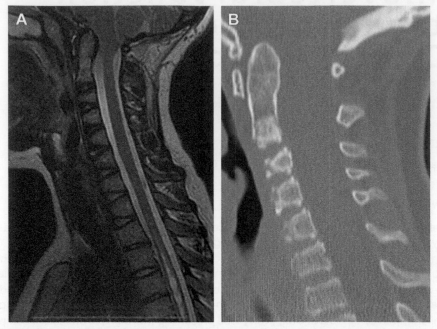

Fig. 1. A 14-year-old girl with known fibroblast growth factor deficiency presented with debilitating occipital headaches. Preoperative MRI (A) and computed tomography scan (B) revealed a CMI with borderline basilar invagination as well as a thoracic syrinx. However, given that she did not have any clinical symptoms or signs concerning for CVJ instability, it was decided to perform a standard posterior fossa suboccipital decompression and C1 laminectomy without dural opening. One year after surgery she remains asymptomatic.

constellation of clinical and radiographic signs, and

2. Discuss the surgical technique for a posterior decompression and stabilization with rigid internal fixation and fusion.

SCOPE OF THE PROBLEM

Regardless of symptom presentation, multiple large studies looking at outcomes after CMI decompression have found posterior fossa decompression alone to successfully alleviate symptoms more than 80% of the time.[1,4–11] Looking at their institutional experience with 500 patients who underwent surgical treatment of pediatric CMI, Tubbs and colleagues[1] report a 3% reoperation rate for continued symptoms or persistent large syringomyelia, with only 4 out of 500 patients requiring transoral odontectomy and occipitocervical fusion.

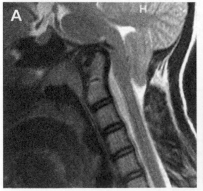
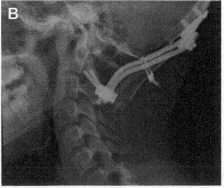

Fig. 2. A 14-year-old girl presented with persistent occipital headaches and dizziness with flexion or extension of her neck. Preoperative MRI (A) demonstrated a CMI with basilar invagination and ventral brainstem compression suggesting CVJ instability. The patient underwent intraoperative reduction followed by suboccipital decompression and occipital-C2 instrumentation and fusion. Postoperative lateral radiograph (B) shows good reduction and alignment. Clinically, she improved considerably with near resolution of her symptoms.

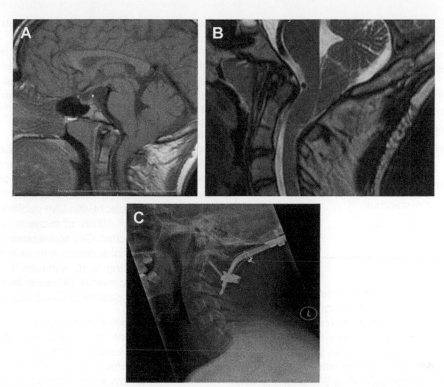

Fig. 3. A 15-year-old boy with CMI (*A*) underwent a posterior fossa decompression at another institution for occipital headaches. Despite initial improvement, his symptoms recurred after several months and he began to develop hypernasal speech, lower cranial nerve palsies, and myelopathy. Subsequent MRI (*B*) showed persistent crowding of the foramen magnum and a retroflexed odontoid with ventral brainstem compression. Because of the previous failed posterior decompression and unsuccessful attempts at preoperative reduction, it was decided to take the patient to the operating room to perform a transnasal resection of the odontoid, a suboccipital decompression with cauterization of the tonsils. (*C*) A postoperative lateral plain film demonstrates good decompression and stabilization.

The prevalence of CVJ instability and the need for stabilization is likely to be skewed by studies from centers known to specialize in CVJ abnormalities. For instance, Brockmeyer[4] found that 10% of patients who underwent surgery for CMI required occipitocervical fusion. Menezes[12] also reported a high incidence of CVJ instability, likely because he mainly focuses on patients who have known CVJ abnormalities, some in conjunction with CMI. In the population at large, however, the coincidence of CVJ instability with CMI is much less frequent.[1,13]

DIAGNOSIS

Defining CVJ instability in the setting of CMI is often challenging. Given the wide variety of causes and radiographic appearances, there is limited consensus among neurosurgeons about the exact clinical and radiographic criteria that should be used when evaluating patients with CMI to determine which patients should undergo CVJ stabilization at the same time as the initial decompression,

or even which patients have a higher likelihood of requiring a stabilization procedure down the line. The diagnosis of CVJ instability should be based both on clinical and radiographic findings.

Clinical Findings

The clinical findings associated with CVJ instability in the setting of CMI are often not distinct from the symptoms attributable to the Chiari malformation alone, or CMI with associated syringomyelia. The most common presenting symptom of CMI is occipital headache, found in 28% to 63% of patients.[1,6,8–11,14–18] Looking at 1700 children presenting with CVJ abnormalities, Menezes found cervical and occipital pain to be present in 85% of subjects. The most common neurologic deficit reported was myelopathy, ranging from monoparesis to quadriparesis, with central cord findings and posterior column dysfunction also commonly seen. Downbeat nystagmus was found to be present more often in patients with CVJ instability and an associated CMI, compared with patients with CVJ instability without a concomitant Chiari (**Box 1**).[19,20]

> **Box 1**
> **Clinical findings suggestive of craniovertebral junction instability in the setting of Chiari I malformation**
>
> - Occipital headache
> - Neck pain
> - Myelopathy
> - Hyperreflexia
> - Central cord syndrome
> - Posterior column dysfunction
> - Downbeat nystagmus
> - Decreased gag reflex
> - Dysphagia

In a large case series of 234 subjects who presented with CMI requiring CVJ stabilization, Fenoy and colleagues[16] found the most common presenting symptom was hyperreflexia in 61% of subjects, followed closely by headache in 58% of subjects. This is in stark contrast to the retrospective series from Tubbs and colleagues[1] of 500 subjects who underwent posterior decompression alone for CMI, very few of whom required further surgical intervention. In this series, lower extremity hyperreflexia was found in only 2.4% of subjects. By far the most frequent presenting symptoms were headache and back pain, seen in 40% of subjects.

Other symptoms that may suggest CVJ instability include a decreased gag response, seen in 39% of subjects who required CVJ fusion in the Fenoy series; upper extremity numbness or paresthesia, in 37% of subjects; and upper-extremity weakness, in 24% of subjects. This again is significantly different from the series from Tubbs and colleagues[1] in which only 8% of subjects presented with upper extremity pain, weakness, or numbness. Fenoy and colleagues[16] also found neck pain, dysphagia, and C2 numbness to each be present in 20% of subjects requiring CVJ fusion, compared with only 4% of subjects who reported dysphagia in the Tubbs and colleagues[1] series.

Radiographic Findings

If a patient presents with a classic CMI, CVJ stability can be assumed, even if there is an associated syringomyelia or scoliosis. In a retrospective study of 210 pediatric subjects who underwent surgical management of Chiari-related malformations, for instance, Brockmeyer[4] found that none of the 173 subjects who had a classic CMI required surgical intervention beyond a suboccipital craniectomy and C1 laminectomy, with or without duraplasty.

There is no radiographic finding that is present in all CMI subjects with CVJ instability. However, several radiographic findings have been associated with CVJ instability and a higher likelihood of requiring CVJ fusion.

Basilar invagination

Basilar invagination, often defined by Chamberlain line or Wackenheim line,[20,21] has been reported in 2% to 38% of CMI patients at the time of initial presentation.[5,13,16,22–26] In a retrospective series of 101 pediatric subjects with CMI published by Bollo and colleagues,[5] 100% of subjects with basilar invagination required CVJ stabilization, compared with only 12.8% of subjects without basilar invagination, suggesting that, although not the only contributor, the presence of basilar invagination itself is highly suggestive of CVJ instability.

Ventral brainstem compression

Traditional means of defining ventral brainstem compression in pediatric patients with CMI relied solely on the presence of basilar invagination. However, it is now known that some patients can have symptomatic ventral compression and CVJ instability in the absence of basilar invagination.

In an effort to better define and assess ventral brainstem compression in patients with CMI, Grabb and colleagues[22] defined a line that extends from the basion to the inferoposterior aspect of the body of C2 (B-C2). They further defined the line as the distance extending perpendicularly from the B-C2 line through the odontoid tip to the ventral dura (pB-C2). Grabb and colleagues[22] found a pB-C2 distance of greater than 9 mm is associated with symptomatic ventral brainstem compression and risk of CVJ instability. Although it has not been validated with large numbers of patients, this distance has subsequently been used as an objective measure of ventral brainstem compression and odontoid retroflexion.

Using a pB-C2 measurement of greater than 5 mm as a cutoff, Brockmeyer[4] found odontoid retroflexion in 20% (32 of 210) of CMI subjects, 13 of whom had successful reduction following CVJ instrumentation and fusion alone. Bollo and colleagues[5] further reported that 74% of subjects who required CVJ fusion had a pB-C2 measurement of greater than or equal to 9 mm, whereas only 24% of subjects who did not require fusion had a pB-C2 measurement of greater than or equal to 9 mm.

Craniocervical angulation

Craniocervical angulation, defined conservatively as a clivoaxial angle (CXA) of less than 125°, has been shown to be a significant predictive factor for requiring CVJ fusion.[5] Defined by Smoker[27] as the angle formed at the intersection of the Wackenheim clivus baseline, a line drawn along the clivus and continued inferiorly into the upper cervical spinal canal, with a line drawn along the posterior surface of the axis body and odontoid process, the craniovertebral, or craniocervical, angle normally ranges from 150° in flexion to 180° in extension. In some CMI patients, this angle may become abnormally acute, with resultant compression of the CVJ. Increased angulation is thought to be indicative of hypermobility, which is associated with CVJ instability.

Chiari 1.5

Chiari 1.5, one of the complex Chiari malformations defined as brainstem herniation through the foramen magnum, has also been reported to be a risk factor for requiring CVJ stabilization and fusion.[4] Bollo and colleagues[5] reported that among 101 children with CMI, 95% (18 out of 19) subjects who required CVJ fusion had Chiari 1.5. In subgroup analyses looking at subjects with Chiari 1.5, CVJ fusion was reported in more than 50% of subjects.[4,5]

Genetic Syndromes

Certain genetic syndromes, namely disorders of connective tissue, may present in conjunction with CMI and are also associated with a predisposition for CVJ instability (**Box 2**). Other genetic

---

Box 2
Genetic syndromes associated with craniovertebral junction instability

- Ehlers-Danlos syndrome
- Mass
- Marfan syndrome
- VACTERL association: Vertebral, anal, cardiac, tracheal, esophageal, renal, and limb anomolies
- Klippel-Feil syndrome
- Achondroplasia
- Down syndrome
- Osteogenesis imperfecta
- Skeletal dysplasias
- Goldenhar syndrome
- Conradi syndrome
- Morquio syndrome
- Hurler syndrome
- Kniest syndrome
- Noonan syndrome

---

syndromes known to be associated with CVJ instability are rarely found in conjunction with CMI. However, when these syndromes do coexist, fusion at the time of the initial decompression may be indicated, given the higher risk for CVJ instability.

Ehlers-Danlos syndrome and other hereditary disorders of connective tissue

One of the defining features of Ehlers-Danlos syndrome and many other hereditary disorders of connective tissue (HDCT) is joint hypermobility, including hypermobility at the occipitoatlantal and atlantoaxial joints. A large study conducted by Milhorat and colleagues[28] looking at 2813 subjects who presented with CMI found a 12.7% coincidence of HDCT and CMI, dramatically higher than the predicted coincidence rate. Of the 357 subjects with CMI and HDCT, the most common connective tissue disorder seen was Ehlers-Danlos syndrome in 149 subjects (42% of subjects with HDCT and Chiari I).

SURGICAL TECHNIQUE

The goals of surgical intervention for patients with CMI and CVJ instability are to relieve compression and stabilize the CVJ. In most cases, both of these goals can be accomplished via a single posterior midline approach. However, in cases with basilar invagination and ventral brainstem compression, preoperative halo traction may be needed to determine if additional anterior decompression will be necessary. This article focuses on posterior decompression and fusion. See the article by Todd C. Hankinson elsewhere in this issue for discussion of anterior approaches.

Preoperative Planning

Imaging

Most children presenting with CMI already have an MRI demonstrating the CMI and the CVJ. If not contraindicated, children suspected of having CVJ instability should have upright cervical spine radiographs with flexion and extension views. If rigid instrumentation and fusion are planned, a computed tomography scan with fine-cut bone windows and 2-dimensional reconstructions is critical to determine if screw placement is technically feasible. Screw lengths, widths, and trajectories should be planned and measured preoperatively using a stereotactic workstation.

Preoperative halo traction or reduction

For children with basilar invagination and ventral brainstem compression, a trial of halo traction should be attempted in most cases to assess reducibility. Although this process can often be difficult, it is important because adequate reduction can obviate a subsequent ventral decompression surgery. Halo pin number and tightness is based on the child's age (**Table 1**), with traction initiated at 3 to 4 lbs and incrementally increased to 7 to 10 lbs if needed.[19] Menezes and Ahmed[19] reported successful reduction with traction in over two-thirds of subjects initially thought to have irreducible lesions. For lesions that are truly irreducible, additional anterior decompression may be required.

Preparation and Positioning

Awake fiber-optic intubation is generally used in most cases of CMI with CVJ instability to minimize the risk of injury. Neuromonitoring with brainstem auditory evoked responses, somatosensory evoked potentials, and motor evoked potentials is routinely used. Consideration should be given to obtaining preposition baseline recordings to insure that no changes occur during positioning. The patient's head should be maintained in neutral position using pins and a skull clamp or by continuing cervical traction. Once positioned, the alignment should be confirmed with lateral fluoroscopy.

If autograft bone is to be used, the preparation and draping should allow for harvesting of posterior iliac crest bone (children >3 years of age) or rib graft.

Surgical Approach

In patients with symptomatic CMI and CVJ instability, the posterior midline approach is the most common approach to decompress the foramen magnum and stabilize the CVJ. In almost all cases, instrumentation and fusion is not needed below C2. The first part of the surgical procedure follows

---

Box 3
Potential complications

Perioperative	Postoperative
• Vertebral artery injury	• Wound infection
• Screw violation of the spinal canal	• Cerebrospinal fluid leak
• Dural tear	• Graft site hematoma
	• Pseudoarthrosis

---

that of a standard posterior fossa decompression for CMI.[29,30] Briefly, a skin incision is made starting from the inion and extending caudally to the spinous process of C3. A midline avascular dissection is carried out, followed by a subperiosteal dissection to expose the inferior occiput, foramen magnum, C1 lamina, and the C2 spinous process and lamina. Care is taken to avoid exposing the full C2-3 joint to prevent possible unintended fusion. A suboccipital craniectomy and C1 laminectomy are then performed. When CVJ stabilization is going to be performed after decompression, strong consideration should be given to performing an expansive duraplasty to maximize the chances for an adequate decompression of the CMI and minimize chances for recurrence. Bone should be preserved to use for autograft for subsequent fusion.

At this point, attention is turned to the CVJ stabilization. The type of construct planned (eg, transarticular screws, C2 pars screws, C1 lateral mass screws, C2 translaminar screws, occipital plate or loop) should be determined preoperatively to insure that the appropriate instrumentation is available. Soft tissue and subperiosteal dissection is continued to expose the medial and lateral surfaces of the C2 pars, the area just superior to the C2-3 joint, and the C1 lateral mass (if needed) to identify entry points for potential screw placement. Fluoroscopy or navigation is then used to assist in screw placement. Percutaneous stab incisions are made for C2 pars screws or C1-C2 transarticular screws if necessary. Once the cervical screws have been placed, an occipital plate is sized and secured using midline screws in the keel

---

Table 1
Halo pin tightness by age

Age (y)	Number of Pins	Tightness (Torque in Inch-Pounds)
1	10	Finger-tightened only
2	8	2
3	8	3
4	8	4
5	8	5
6	8	6
>6	4	8

Data from Hickman Z, McDowell M, Anderson RC. Principles of pediatric spinal column trauma. In: Albright AL, Pollack I, Adelson RD, editors. Principles and practice of pediatric neurosurgery. 3rd edition. New York: Thieme; 2014. p. 6040–799.

Box 4
Suggested pain-control regimen

• Toradol 0.5 mg/kg intravenous (IV) every 6 hours

• Valium 0.1 mg/kg IV every 6 hours

• Morphine 0.1 mg/kg every 3 hours when necessary for breakthrough pain

Table 2
Clinical results in the literature

Author (year)	Total Number of Subjects	Intervention	Main Findings
Bollo et al,[5] 2012	101	PFD (82) PFD + craniovertebral fusion (19)	Multivariate analysis: factors demonstrating significantly increased risk of requiring fusion included basilar invagination, CM 1.5, and CXA <125
Brockmeyer,[4] 2011	210	PFD (210, 100%) PFD + craniovertebral fusion (21, 10%) PFD + transoral odontoid resection (10, 4%)	0 SBs w classic CMI required further surgical intervention 56% SBs w Chiari 1.5 underwent craniovertebral fusion 22% SBs underwent odontoid resection 21 SBs underwent craniovertebral fusion 13 SBs had successful reduction of a retroflexed odontoid w posterior instrumentation and fusion alone
Tubbs et al,[1] 2011	500	PFD + D (499) PFD – D (1)	15 SBs (3%) required reoperation for persistent syringomyelia or HA 4 SBs subsequently developed SXs referable to brainstem compression and underwent transoral odontectomy occipitocervical fusion All 4 SBs had severe odontoid retroflexion w ventral brainstem compression 1 SB had significant basilar invagination
Fenoy et al,[16] 2008	234	Dorsal CVJ fusion (235, 100%) + Dorsal PFD (170, 73%) + Combined dorsal PFD and ventral brainstem decompression (51, 22%)	Most common presenting SXs associated with CVJ instability included hyperreflexia, HA, decreased gag reflex, UE numbness or paresthesia, UE weakness, neck pain, dysphagia, and C2 numbness
Grabb et al,[22] 1999	34	PFD + D (34, 100%) 4 SBs underwent halo ring traction before surgery secondary to VBSC 3 of the 4 SBs were treated w posterior decompression and craniovertebral fusion and instrumentation in mild extension 1 SB underwent a transoral odontoidectomy before the posterior procedure	All SBs w pB-C2 <9 mm underwent only PFD w good clinical results 7 SBs w pB-C2 ≥9 underwent only PFD with good clinical results 3 SBs underwent initial posterior decompression and fusion: 1 deteriorated postoperatively w new-onset lower CN dysfunction secondary to ongoing ventral compression, necessitating transoral odontoidectomy

Abbreviations: CM, Chiari malformation; CN, cranial nerve; D, duraplasty; HA, headache; PFD, posterior fossa decompression; SB, subject; SX, symptom; UE, upper extremity; VBSC, ventral brainstem compression; w, with.
Data from Refs.[1,4,5,16,22]

approximately 1 cm above the craniectomy site to allow adequate space for a midline fusion mass. Rods are then cut and bent to size, top loaded in the screws bilaterally, and the set screws are locked in place. Alternatively, a single-piece occipital cervical loop can be used. If a structural autograft is desired, bone is harvested from either the posterior iliac crest or posterior rib and measured and cut to fit in the space from the inferior aspect of the occipital plate to the top of the C2 spinous process. The superior edge of the C2 lamina is drilled away, leaving a shelf ventrally to prevent telescoping of the graft into the spinal canal. The wound is irrigated and hemostasis is achieved. The bone is then decorticated and the graft is placed. Titanium cables can be used around the rods and graft to secure the graft and create a compressive force to facilitate bone fusion. Local autograft and graft extenders are then used, if desired, to fill in the areas surrounding the graft. Meticulous hemostasis is achieved, and the muscle, fascia, and subcutaneous tissues are closed in layers. **Box 3** presents potential perioperative and postoperative complications.

Immediate Postoperative Care

Postoperatively, antibiotics are continued for 24 hours. Pain is typically well controlled with the combination of intravenous Toradol and Valium, with morphine reserved for breakthrough pain (**Box 4**). After 24 to 48 hours, most patients can be transitioned to oral pain medications in preparation for discharge. A halo vest is generally not necessary postoperatively but patients are encouraged to wear a hard cervical collar for 4 to 6 weeks. Upright anteroposterior and lateral radiographs are generally obtained postoperatively, at 3 to 4 months, 1 year, and 2 years follow-up.

DISCUSSION

It is important to keep in mind that CVJ instability in the setting of CMI is uncommon and most patients, even those with signs of brainstem compression at the time of initial presentation, will improve with a standard posterior fossa decompression. However, there are a constellation of signs and symptoms that, if taken together, are highly suggestive of CVJ instability.

The most suggestive clinical findings associated with CVJ instability in the setting of CMI seem to be myelopathy and hyperreflexia (**Table 2**). Patients with CVJ instability also have a higher incidence of decreased gag reflex, dysphasia, central cord syndrome, posterior column dysfunction, and downbeat nystagmus.

Several radiographic findings have been identified that are suggestive of CVJ instability. These include traditional measurements of basilar invagination, defined by Chamberlain line or Wackenheim line; signs of ventral brainstem compression, defined by a pB-C2 measurement of greater than or equal to 9 mm; a CXA of less than 125°; and Chiari 1.5 malformation. However, there is no single radiographic finding that is in itself diagnostic of CVJ instability. In patients with basilar invagination and ventral brainstem compression, a preoperative trial of traction is often necessary to determine if the lesion is reducible, in which case it can be addressed with a posterior decompression and stabilization alone. Otherwise, additional anterior decompression may be necessary to adequately address the brainstem compression and alleviate symptoms.

In patients with CMI and CVJ instability, symptoms often do not improve, and may even worsen, following posterior decompression without additional anterior decompression and/or occipital cervical stabilization, making continued evaluation paramount in the proper management of these patients.

REFERENCES

1. Tubbs RS, Beckman J, Naftel RP, et al. Institutional experience with 500 cases of surgically treated pediatric Chiari malformation Type I. J Neurosurg Pediatr 2011;7(3):248–56.
2. Anderson RC, Dowling KC, Feldstein NA, et al. Chiari I malformation: potential role for intraoperative electrophysiologic monitoring. J Clin Neurophysiol 2003;20(1):65–72.
3. Anderson RC, Emerson RG, Dowling KC, et al. Improvement in brainstem auditory evoked potentials after suboccipital decompression in patients with chiari I malformations. J Neurosurg 2003; 98(3):459–64.
4. Brockmeyer DL. The complex Chiari: issues and management strategies. Neurol Sci 2011;32(Suppl 3):S345–7.
5. Bollo RJ, Riva-Cambrin J, Brockmeyer MM, et al. Complex Chiari malformations in children: an analysis of preoperative risk factors for occipitocervical fusion. J Neurosurg Pediatr 2012;10(2):134–41.
6. Tubbs RS, McGirt MJ, Oakes WJ. Surgical experience in 130 pediatric patients with Chiari I malformations. J Neurosurg 2003;99(2):291–6.
7. Albert GW, Menezes AH, Hansen DR, et al. Chiari malformation Type I in children younger than age 6 years: presentation and surgical outcome. J Neurosurg Pediatr 2010;5(6):554–61.
8. Alzate JC, Kothbauer KF, Jallo GI, et al. Treatment of Chiari I malformation in patients with and without

syringomyelia: a consecutive series of 66 cases. Neurosurg Focus 2001;11(1):E3.

9. Park JK, Gleason PL, Madsen JR, et al. Presentation and management of Chiari I malformation in children. Pediatr Neurosurg 1997;26(4):190–6.

10. Genitori L, Peretta P, Nurisso C, et al. Chiari type I anomalies in children and adolescents: minimally invasive management in a series of 53 cases. Childs Nerv Syst 2000;16(10–11):707–18.

11. Krieger MD, McComb JG, Levy ML. Toward a simpler surgical management of Chiari I malformation in a pediatric population. Pediatr Neurosurg 1999;30(3):113–21.

12. Menezes AH. Craniovertebral junction abnormalities with hindbrain herniation and syringomyelia: regression of syringomyelia after removal of ventral craniovertebral junction compression. J Neurosurg 2012; 116(2):301–9.

13. Milhorat TH, Chou MW, Trinidad EM, et al. Chiari I malformation redefined: clinical and radiographic findings for 364 symptomatic patients. Neurosurgery 1999;44(5):1005–17.

14. Alden TD, Ojemann JG, Park TS. Surgical treatment of Chiari I malformation: indications and approaches. Neurosurg Focus 2001;11(1):E2.

15. Cheng JS, Nash J, Meyer GA. Chiari type I malformation revisited: diagnosis and treatment. Neurologist 2002;8(6):357–62.

16. Fenoy AJ, Menezes AH, Fenoy KA. Craniocervical junction fusions in patients with hindbrain herniation and syringohydromyelia. J Neurosurg Spine 2008; 9(1):1–9.

17. Navarro R, Olavarria G, Seshadri R, et al. Surgical results of posterior fossa decompression for patients with Chiari I malformation. Childs Nerv Syst 2004; 20(5):349–56.

18. Pascual J, Oterino A, Berciano J. Headache in type I Chiari malformation. Neurology 1992;42(8):1519–21.

19. Menezes AH, Ahmed R. Craniovertebral Junction. Congenital and Developmental Spinal Disorders. 342–56.

20. Menezes AH. Craniovertebral junction abnormalities. In: Albright A, Pollack I, Adelson P, editors. Principles and practice of pediatric neurosurgery, vol. III. New York: Thieme Medical Publishers; 2008. p. 395–414.

21. Wackenheim A. Radiologic diagnosis of congenital forms, intermittent forms and progressive forms of stenosis of the spinal canal at the level of the atlas. Acta Radiol Diagn (Stockh) 1969;9:759–68 [in French].

22. Grabb PA, Mapstone TB, Oakes WJ. Ventral brain stem compression in pediatric and young adult patients with Chiari I malformations. Neurosurgery 1999;44(3):520–7 [discussion: 527–8].

23. Dyste GN, Menezes AH. Presentation and management of pediatric Chiari malformations without myelodysplasia. Neurosurgery 1988;23(5):589–97.

24. Ladner TR, Dewan MC, Day MA, et al. Evaluating the relationship of the pB-C2 line to clinical outcomes in a 15-year single-center cohort of pediatric Chiari I malformation. J Neurosurg Pediatr 2015;15(2):178–88.

25. Goel A, Bhatjiwale M, Desai K. Basilar invagination: a study based on 190 surgically treated patients. J Neurosurg 1998;88(6):962–8.

26. Menezes AH, Fenoy KA. Remnants of occipital vertebrae: proatlas segmentation abnormalities. Neurosurgery 2009;64(5):945–53 [discussion: 954].

27. Smoker WR. Craniovertebral junction: normal anatomy, craniometry, and congenital anomalies. Radiographics 1994;14(2):255–77.

28. Milhorat TH, Bolognese PA, Nishikawa M, et al. Syndrome of occipitoatlantoaxial hypermobility, cranial settling, and chiari malformation type I in patients with hereditary disorders of connective tissue. J Neurosurg Spine 2007;7(6):601–9.

29. Tyler-Kabara EC, Oakes WJ. Chiari malformations and syringohydromyelia. In: Goodrich JT, editor. Neurosurgical operative atlas: pediatric neurosurgery. 2nd edition. New York: Thieme; 2008. p. 7–12.

30. Tubbs RS, Griessenauer CJ, Oakes WJ. Chiari malformations. In: Albright AL, Pollack IF, Adelson PD, editors. Principles and practice of pediatric neurosurgery. 3rd edition. New York: Thieme; 2015. p. 192–204.

Ventral Decompression in Chiari Malformation, Basilar Invagination, and Related Disorders

Thomas Ridder, MD[a],*, Richard C.E. Anderson, MD[b],
Todd C. Hankinson, MD[a,c]

KEYWORDS

- Ventral brainstem compression • Chiari malformation, type I (CM-I) • Basilar invagination • pB-C2
- Transoral and transnasal approaches

KEY POINTS

- Ventral brainstem compression (VBSC) is an uncommon clinical diagnosis seen by pediatric neurosurgeons and associated with Chiari malformation, type I (CM-I).
- Presenting clinical symptoms often include headaches, lower cranial neuropathies, myelopathy, central sleep apnea, ataxia, and nystagmus.
- When ventral decompression is required, both open and endoscopic transoral/transnasal approaches are highly effective.

INTRODUCTION

This article summarizes the clinical manifestations and surgical options for the treatment of patients who present with VBSC in the context of CM-I or other craniovertebral junction (CVJ) anomalies.[1]

VENTRAL BRAINSTEM DECOMPRESSION
Background

Prior to the development of modern imaging and operative techniques, a diagnosis of VBSC was typically made post mortem.[2] The most common causes of VBSC at the CVJ include inflammatory conditions, such as rheumatoid arthritis; trauma; and tumors. In some cases, VBSC is associated with CM-I. Efforts to surgically treat VBSC associated with CM-I began with posterior decompression with or without fusion and advanced to include direct ventral decompression.[3] These techniques were pioneered by surgeons, such as

Kanavel, who, in 1917, used the transoral route to remove a bullet lodged between the atlas and clivus.[4] Advances in neuroimaging and surgical technique (eg, transnasal endoscopy) have broadened the armamentarium for approaches to these usually complex problems. Factors that influence the specific surgical treatment include

1. Patient age
2. Symptomatology
3. Etiology of the pathologic process
4. Reducibility of the compressive lesion.

Ventral Brainstem Compression in Chiari Malformation, Type I

Although CM-I has been recognized as a common entity, identified in 1% to 5% of all patients undergoing head and cervical MRIs,[5] the identification of VBSC is less common.[3,5] In a review of 364 symptomatic adults with CM-I, however, Milhorat and

[a] Children's Hospital Colorado, 13123 East 16th Avenue, Aurora, CO 80045, USA; [b] Department of Neurosurgery, Columbia University Medical Center, New York, NY 10032, USA; [c] Department of Neurosurgery, University of Colorado Anschutz Medical Campus, Aurora, CO 80045, USA
* Corresponding author.
E-mail address: thomas.ridder@childrenscolorado.org

Neurosurg Clin N Am 26 (2015) 571–578
http://dx.doi.org/10.1016/j.nec.2015.06.011
1042-3680/15/$ – see front matter © 2015 Elsevier Inc. All rights reserved.

colleagues[6,7] identified an abnormally retroflexed odontoid process in 26% and basilar invagination (BI) in 12%.[8] In their study of 38 patients, Grabb and colleagues[9,10] quantified the extent of VBSC in 40 pediatric and young adult patients through measurement of a line perpendicular to the basion-C2 line (B-C2), termed the *pB-C2* (**Fig. 1**). The group found that all patients with a pB-C2 measurement of less than 9 mm were treated successfully with posterior fossa decompression alone, despite the presence of VBSC on subjective evaluation. A subset of patients with pB-C2 measurements greater than 9 mm required occipitocervical stabilization with or without ventral decompression in addition to posterior fossa decompression. These investigators also noted that pB-C2 did not increase with age. Ladner and colleagues[11–14] described ventral canal encroachment in a pediatric population as a pB-C2 greater than 3 mm. In their series, only 1.3%

of patients demonstrated a pB-C2 greater than 9 mm and none required ventral decompression.

Incidence of Ventral Brainstem Compression in Basilar Invagination and Related Disorders

BI, or basilar impression, is an uncommon condition in the general population but it may be identified in as many 25% to 35% patients with CM-I.[15] BI is most commonly a developmental anomaly of the CVJ in which the odontoid process prolapses into or through the foramen magnum. It is associated with several underlying congenital, metabolic, and inflammatory conditions (**Box 1**). BI often coexists with osseous anomalies of the CVJ, including atlanto-occipital assimilation; incomplete ring of C1; and hypoplasia of the basiocciput, occipital condyles, and atlas.[15]

DIAGNOSIS OF VENTRAL BRAINSTEM COMPRESSION
Clinical Examination

In the context of CM-I, patients with VBSC may present with the classic signs and symptoms of reversible occipitocervical headache or neck pain. The presentation may be insidious or rapid, and false localizing signs may be present. There are numerous studies discussing the spectrum of symptoms encountered in CM-I but also VBSC.[16–22] These symptoms can range from a mild basilar headache to progressive cranial neuropathies and wheelchair dependence. As recently described by Menezes,[23] however, this population is more likely to also demonstrate long tract signs, myelopathy, brainstem dysfunction, and lower cranial nerve abnormalities. In their series, 3 of 84 patients (3.6%) suffered facial pain and another 6 (7.1%) experienced facial hypalgesia. Urinary frequency and incontinence were present in 14 of 84 patients (16.7%). **Box 2** shows typical clinical signs/symptoms of VBSC associated with CVJ anomalies.

Radiographic Findings

Both pediatric and adult patients who present with signs/symptoms consistent with CM-I or VBSC should be evaluated with MRI. CM-I is diagnosed when the cerebellar tonsils herniate greater than or equal to 5 mm below the level of McRae line (drawn from the basion to the opisthion). When CM-I is identified, imaging of the entire spinal cord should be reviewed for the presence of syringomyelia. BI has been assessed through several measures, including the relationship of the odontoid tip to Chamberlain line (drawn from the posterior hard palate to the opisthion), McRae line,

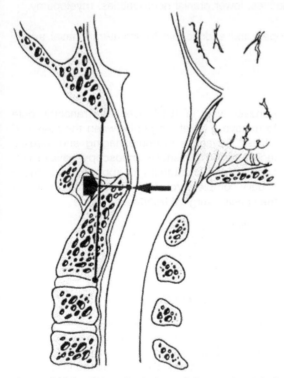

Fig. 1. Sketch of a sagittal view of the craniocervical junction showing the B-C2 line, drawn from the basion to the inferoposterior aspect of the C2 body, and a line perpendicular to this line, pB-C2, drawn through the odontoid tip to the ventral cervicomedullary dura. The distance of pB-C2 is then measured in millimeters between the thick and the thin *arrows*. (*From* Grabb PA, Mapstone TB, Oakes WJ. Ventral brain stem compression in pediatric and young adult patients with Chiari I malformations. Neurosurgery 1999;44(3):522 [discussion: 527–8]; with permission.)

Box 1
Classification of craniovertebral junction anomalies associated with ventral brainstem compression

I. Congenital malformations of occipital sclerotome, atlas, and/or axis

A. Occipital sclerotome malformations—proatlas remnants, clivus segmentations, condylar hypoplasia, atlas assimilation

B. Atlas malformations—bifid atlas, assimilation, fusions, absent arches

C. Axis malformations—segmentation defects, odontoid dysplasias

II. Developmental and acquired malformations

A. Malformations at foramen magnum

1. BI—osteogenesis imperfecta, hypophosphatemic rickets, Paget disease, hyperparathyroidism, Klippel-Feil syndrome, Hajdu-Cheney syndrome

2. Stenosis at foramen magnum—achondroplasia, paramesial invagination

B. Disorders leading to atlantoaxial instability

1. Infections—tuberculosis

2. Down syndrome

3. Trauma

4. Inflammatory—regional ileitis, reiter syndrome, juvenile rheumatoid arthritis, eosinophilic granuloma

5. Malignancy—osteoblastoma, chordoma

Adapted from Menezes AH. Craniovertebral junction database analysis: incidence, classification, presentation, and treatment algorithms. Childs Nerv Syst 2008;24(10):1104; with permission.

Wackenheim clival canal line (drawn along the sagittal plane of the clivus and extending into the cervical canal), the length of the clivus (measured from the top of the dorsum sellae to the basion), the anteroposterior width of the foramen magnum, and the basal angle (**Fig. 2**).[23,24]

Box 2
Signs and symptoms of craniovertebral anomalies associated with ventral brainstem compression

Posterior occipital headache or neck pain

Myelopathy or quadraparesis

Basilar migraines

Lower cranial neuropathies (eg, dysphagia, aspiration pneumonia, and diminished gag reflex)

Facial pain

Urinary frequency or incontinence

Ataxia

Nystagmus (downbeat and lateral gaze)

Central sleep apnea

Sensory disturbances (posterior column dysfunction)

Hearing loss or tinnitus

In the presence of VBSC, additional imaging should include flexion/extension occipitocervical radiographs to evaluate for pathologic motion. Noncontrast CT better defines the osseous anatomy and should be evaluated if posterior instrumentation is planned. In addition, the vascular imaging, either with MRI or CT, should be strongly considered prior to surgical intervention, because the course of the vertebral arteries is commonly anomalous in the context of VBSC.

As described by Grabb and colleagues,[9] using a midsagittal MRI, the B-C2 can be drawn from the basion to the inferoposterior aspect of the C2 body. The distance of the longest pB-C2 from the B-C2 line through the odontoid to the ventral dura, may serve as an objective measurement of encroachment by the odontoid and any investing tissues into the foramen magnum or rostral spinal canal (see **Fig. 2**).[9]

TREATMENT OF VENTRAL BRAINSTEM COMPRESSION IN THE CONTEXT OF CHIARI MALFORMATION, TYPE I
Nonoperative (Conservative)

In both the pediatric and adult populations, treatment of CM-I is predicated on the presence of signs or symptoms that can be clearly attributed to the lesion. As such, in the absence of these,

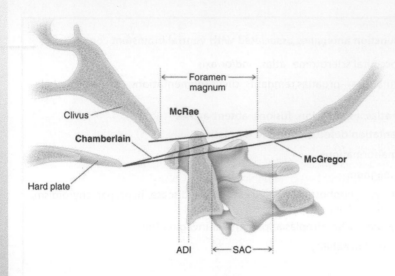

Fig. 2. Commonly assessed craniovertebral metrics. (*From* Herring JA. Tachdjian's pediatric orthopaedics. 5th edition. Elsevier; 2013; with permission.)

careful clinical monitoring may be considered even in the presence of some degree VBSC. In cases of conservative management considered, the authors complete a careful neurologic examination that includes attempts to elicit signs/symptoms of brainstem compression throughout the cervical range of motion. In the absence of these, the occipitocervical junction is evaluated with dynamic radiographs. The frequency of radiographic follow-up should be determined on a case-by-case basis.

Surgical Treatment

Goals of surgery

The goal of VBSC is to relieve pressure on the brainstem and upper spinal cord. In the absence of existing craniocervical instability, operative decompression in the context of CM-I or BI almost always results in instability, mandating adjunctive operative posterior stabilization.

Ventral approaches to craniocervical junction

The most common approaches to the ventral CVJ in the context of CM-I include open transoral and endoscopic transnasal routes.

Open transoral approach The standard transoral approach provides midline exposure of the inferior one-third of the clivus, ventral CVJ, and the C1–C2 complex. It provides a direct extradural exposure that does not require brain retraction. The transoral approach is associated with morbidity based on the need for prolonged retraction of the tongue, which results in subsequent airway edema, often requiring intubation and tube feeding for several days after surgery.

Positioning and application of transoral retractor system After oral fiberoptic intubation, the head is secured in pin fixation to allow for intraoperative stereotaxis (which the authors prefer). The patient is positioned supine with the head in slight extension, facilitating a direct line of sight to the CVJ. Topical corticosteroid cream can be applied to the tongue to reduce postoperative tongue swelling. The transoral retractor system (eg, Spetzler-Sonntag or Dingman) is selected based on surgeon preference. The uvula and soft palate can be retracted using a suture or retractor blade and rarely need to be divided to gain exposure. The patient's tongue can be retracted inferiorly using a wide and rigid retractor blade. The endotracheal tube can be placed under the tongue retractor or, preferably, along the side of the mouth to reduce tongue compression. Guards may be used to protect the upper teeth. Lateral retractors move the oral-pharyngeal soft tissues laterally. After the retractor system is in place, it is important to carefully inspect the tongue to confirm that it is free from compression between the retractor blade and the teeth. Failure to recognize this compression can result in necrosis or swelling of the tongue. After final positioning of the retractors, the mouth, oropharynx, and retractors are prepped with Betadine solution. In these cases, the surgeon is positioned at the head of the patient and uses an operating microscope.

Incision and muscle dissection The posterior pharyngeal wall can be infiltrated with 0.5% lidocaine with 1:200,000 epinephrine, per surgeon preference. The anterior tubercle of C1 is usually palpable but can be reliably identified using stereotaxis. The posterior pharyngeal mucosa can be opened with a blade or shielded monopolar cautery on low power. It is incised longitudinally in the midline and dissection is carried through the midline raphe between the pharyngeal muscles and to the anterior tubercle through the anterior longitudinal ligament, using palpation and stereotaxis to verify the appropriate trajectory. Subperiosteal monopolar dissection minimizes bleeding and allows retraction of the longus capitis muscles, revealing the C1 arch. The authors then extend the exposure superiorly and inferiorly, to expose the inferior clivus and C2 body.

Removal of C1 arch and odontoidectomy Using a high-speed drill and rongeurs under magnification, the authors resect the anterior arch of C1 to a width just beyond the lateral extent of the dens. In some cases, there may be a substantial soft tissue pannus between the resected anterior arch and the ventral aspect of the dens. This tissue is removed using rongeurs. The borders of the dens are defined and ligamentous attachments are released, taking special care to free the apical and alar ligaments. The dens is drilled carefully until only a thin rim of dorsal cortical bone remains. This is carefully elevated off the underlying soft tissues or dura using angled curettes, rongeurs, or a diamond tip burr. The superior cap of the dens must be mobilized and resected, which can be challenging if it is free-floating after release from the inferior portion of the dens. After removal of the odontoid tip, the transverse ligament, tectorial membrane, and any pannus may be removed. If necessary, the inferior clivus maybe resected using a high-speed drill, curettes, and rongeurs. The underlying dura or posterior longitudinal ligament should be observed to be pulsatile and should be palpated to verify adequate decompression.

Closure Multiple closure techniques have been described after transoral odontoidectomy.[4,25–27] Both the muscle and mucosal layers may be reapproximated using 3-0 Vicryl suture, taking care to avoid strangulation of the mucosal tissue. In the absence of cerebrospinal fluid (CSF) leak, fibrin glue may not be necessary. Obtaining a watertight dural closure may be difficult and can be improved with fibrin glue (Tisseel) or polyethylene glycol dural sealant (DuraSeal) and placement of lumbar drain for CSF diversion.

Endoscopic transnasal or transoral approach The development of experience using the endoscopic transnasal approach to the sellar region led to the application of both transoral and transnasal endoscopic approaches to the CVJ (**Table 1**). A cadaveric study using a transoral approach demonstrated superior exposure using an endoscopic approach, when compared with an open microscopic approach.[28]

The endoscopic transnasal approach is the authors' preferred means of accessing the odontoid, when a patient's anatomy allows adequate exposure. This approach not only offers excellent visualization but also minimizes trauma to the oropharynx, thereby facilitating early extubation and oral nutrition.

Positioning and approach As with the transoral microscopic approach, the patient is positioned supine with slight extension in a rigid headholder to allow for stereotactic navigation. The authors' preference is to rotate the head slightly toward the operating surgeon, who stands on the patient's right side. Although turbinate resection may be needed in young patients, lateralization of the inferior turbinates provides sufficient space for the surgeon to maneuver instruments in older children and adults. The sphenoid sinus does not need to be entered. A posterior nasal septectomy enlarges the choana to maximize exposure and the trajectory is confirmed with stereotactic navigation. Adenoidectomy is performed using electrocautery or a microdébrider. The posterior nasopharynx is opened in a linear fashion from the clivus to the

---

Table 1
Advantages/disadvantages of transoral and transnasal approaches to the ventral craniocervical junction

Approach	Advantages	Disadvantages
Transoral	Direct visualization of CVJ	Higher risk of contamination if dural opening Dysphagia, intubation, and nasogastric tube expected postoperatively Must retract uvula/palate
Transnasal	Excellent visualization Minimizes trauma to oropharynx Earlier extubation and oral nutrition	Limited by size of nares Trajectory sometimes limited by palate

level of the C2 vertebral body, with the lateral margins just medial to the tori of the eustachian tubes. The longus colli and capitis muscles are mobilized laterally and the anterior tubercle of C1 is identified. Ventral decompression is then completed using the same steps, as described previously, through an open transoral approach. The anterior ring of C1 and dens removal is used, as described previously.

Closure In most cases, the dura remains intact after ventral decompression. This facilitates closure, which can include reapproximation of the mucosal layers supported by a layer of fibrin glue. If the dura is violated, then the authors reconstruct the defect in the same manner as with endonasal transsphenoidal procedures that include a substantial dural defect. This includes positioning a layer of synthetic dural graft inside the defect, followed by a nasal septal flap, tisseal, and autologous fat graft. Whether or not a dural defect is encountered, absorbable nasal packs are placed to facilitate healing of the denuded nasal mucosa.

Transmaxillary and high cervical retropharyngeal approaches Historically, transmaxillary approaches provided access to lesions requiring greater superior exposure than that offered with a transoral approach. When combined with maxillotomies, the transoral approach can expose the majority of the clivus and upper cervical spine. This method, however, carries a greater risk of wound infection and of swallowing and speech difficulties than less aggressive approaches. In the context of CM-I with VBSC, there is currently little need for transmaxillary approaches. High cervical retropharyngeal approaches have never been published for treatment of VBSC from CM-I. They have been successfully applied to approach the CVJ in the context of chordomas with lateral and caudal extension.[27]

Sequence of procedures

For a majority of patients with CM-I, posterior decompression adequately treats the presenting symptoms and radiographic compression. Although posterior instrumented fusion is not required in many cases where VBSC is evident,[9] it often alleviates or prevents symptoms related to VBSC without the need for direct ventral decompression. The role of prefusion traction to reduce BI is assessed on a case-by-case basis. As such, the authors do not generally undertake ventral decompression prior to posterior occipitocervical fusion. This decision, however, is also made on an individual basis. When ventral decompression is definitively required, positioning for a transoral approach may be limited by a posterior

fusion and some surgeons may, therefore, prefer to complete the ventral decompression first. When an endoscopic transnasal approach is planned, a preexisting occipitocervical fusion does not substantially have an impact on patient positioning.

Although no specific measurement or group of measures has been shown to predict the need for ventral decompression, a detailed understanding of a patient's craniovertebral anatomy as well as the use of indices, such as the pB-C2 line, can assist the with decisionmaking regarding patients with VBSC.

Case example A 12-year-old boy with osteogenesis imperfecta presented with progressive quadriparesis, vocal cord paralysis, and respiratory insufficiency. Radiographic imaging confirmed the diagnosis of CM- I with BI and VBSC (**Fig. 3**). Initial attempts at reduction failed. Suboccipital craniectomy and C-1 laminectomy with cerebellar tonsil reduction and expansive duraplasty were undertaken. These were supplemented with an occiput–C2 instrumented fusion. The patient recovered well and was discharged home with independent airway control and stable quadriparesis and at his baseline regarding speech and swallowing function. Five months later, the patient presented to an outside institution with vocal cord paralysis, progressive weakness, anisocoria, and central apnea requiring intubation. CT and MRI demonstrated anterior

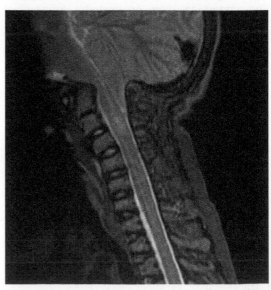

Fig. 3. Sagittal T2-weighted MRI scan at presentation, demonstrating CM-I with BI and substantial VBSC. There is no syringomyelia.

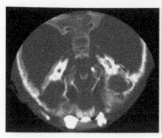
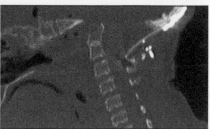

Fig. 4. Postoperative images after the first transnasal odontoidectomy. (*Left*) Axial CT scan demonstrating partial resection of the dens at the level of the clivus. (*Right*) Sagittal CT scan demonstrating partial resection of the superior odontoid process. (*From* Hickman ZL, McDowell MM, Barton SM, et al. Transnasal endoscopic approach to the pediatric CVJ and rostral cervical spine: case series and literature review. Neurosurg Focus 2013;35(2):E14; with permission.)

cervicomedullary compression and upward mass effect on the midbrain due to a retroflexed odontoid process. Decompression was planned via an endoscopic transnasal approach. After what seemed a successful initial decompression, the patient had an improvement in speech and motor strength but remained ventilator dependent, prompting imaging that demonstrated incomplete odontoid resection (**Fig. 4**). He was, therefore, taken back for repeat odontoidectomy, which was confirmed with CT imaging prior to the reversal of general anesthesia.

The patient did well after his second surgery with resumption of oral feedings with gastrostomy tube supplementation on postoperative day 1. His neurologic examination continued to improve and he had daytime ventilator independence by postoperative day 10. Postoperative MRI demonstrated mild to moderate cervicomedullary edema. At 9 months after his second surgery, the patient had been successfully weaned off all mechanical ventilation. Repeat imaging at that time demonstrated a stable decompression of the cervicomedullary junction, a solid occiput–C2 fusion, and a dramatic reduction of the previously noted cervicomedullary swelling (**Fig. 5**).

SUMMARY

Although VBSC is an uncommon neurosurgical problem, it is an important diagnosis to consider and manage appropriately. Neurologic sequelae can be life threatening, and permanent injury is associated with a high degree of morbidity. Signs and symptoms include limited range of motion, hearing loss, functional decline, aspiration pneumonia, and central apnea. When VBSC is associated with CM-I, posterior decompression with or without instrumented fusion often stabilizes or improves symptoms related to brainstem compression. When ventral decompression is required, transoral and transnasal approaches have been shown to provide excellent visualization of the CVJ and are associated with good clinical outcomes.

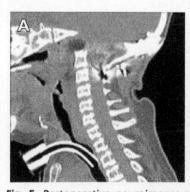
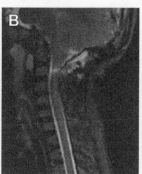
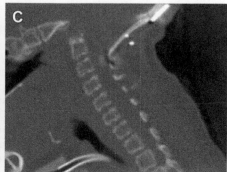

Fig. 5. Postoperative neuroimages after the second transnasal odontoidectomy. (*A*) Sagittal CT scan demonstrating complete resection of the odontoid. (*B*) Follow-up sagittal T2-weighted MRI demonstrating reduced cervicomedullary edema and possible chronic gliosis. (*C*) Follow-up sagittal CT scan demonstrating the long-term maintenance of spinal alignment and decompression. (*From* Hickman ZL, McDowell MM, Barton SM, et al. Transnasal endoscopic approach to the pediatric CVJ and rostral cervical spine: case series and literature review. Neurosurg Focus 2013;35(2):E14; with permission.)

REFERENCES

1. Bhangoo RS, Crockard HA. Transmaxillary anterior decompression in patients with severe basilar impression. Clin Orthop 1999;359:115–25.
2. DeBarros MC, Farais W, Ataide L, et al. Basilar impression and Arnold-Chiari malformation: a study of 66 cases. J Neurol Neurosurg Psychiatry 1968; 31:596–605.
3. Dyste GN, Menezes AH. Presentation and management of pediatric Chiari malformations without myelodysplasia. Neurosurgery 1988;23:589–97.
4. Choi D, Crockard HA. Evolution of transoral surgery: three decades of change in patients, pathologies, and indications. Neurosurgery 2013;73(2):296–303 [discussion: 303–4].
5. Elster AD, Chen MY. Chiari I malformations: clinical and radiologic reappraisal. Radiology 1992;183: 347–53.
6. Milhorat TH, Chou MW, Trinidad EM, et al. Chiari I malformation redefined: clinical and radiographic findings for 364 symptomatic patients. Neurosurgery 1999;44:1005–17.
7. Pillai P, Baig MN, Karas CS, et al. Endoscopic image-guided transoral approach to the craniovertebral junction: an anatomic study comparing surgical exposure and surgical freedom obtained with the endoscope and the operating microscope. Neurosurgery 2009;64(5 Suppl 2):437–42 [discussion: 442–4].
8. Menezes AH. Craniovertebral junction abnormalities with hindbrain herniation and syringomyelia: regression of syringomyelia after removal of ventral craniovertebral junction compression. J Neurosurg 2012; 116(2):301–9.
9. Grabb PA, Mapstone TB, Oakes WJ. Ventral brain stem compression in pediatric and young adult patients with Chiari I malformations. Neurosurgery 1999;44(3):520–7 [discussion: 527–8].
10. Greenberg JK, Yarbrough CK, Radmanesh A, et al. The Chiari severity index: a preoperative grading system for chiari malformation type 1. Neurosurgery 2015;76(3):279–85.
11. Ladner TR, Dewan MC, Day MA, et al. Evaluating the relationship of the pB-C2 line to clinical outcomes in a 15-year single-center cohort of pediatric Chiari I malformation. J Neurosurg Pediatr 2015; 15(2):178–88.
12. Lee MC, Ryu SI, Rhoton AL, et al. Transmaxillary approach to the clivus and upper cervical spine. In: Surgical anatomy and techniques of the spine. 1st edition. Philadelphia: Elsevier; 2006. p. 13–21.
13. List CF. Neurologic syndromes accompanying developmental anomalies of occipital bone, atlas and axis. Arch Neurol Psychiatry 1941;45:577–616.
14. Liu JK, Couldwell WT, Apfelbaum RI. Transoral approach and extended modifications for lesions of the ventral foramen magnum and craniovertebral junction. Skull Base 2008;18(3):151–66.
15. Smith JS, Shaffrey CI, Abel MF, et al. Basilar invagination. Neurosurgery 2010;66(3 Suppl):39–47.
16. Greenlee JDW, Donovan KA, Hasan DM, et al. Chiari I malformation in the very young child: the spectrum of presentations and experience in 31 children under age 6 years. Pediatrics 2002;110(6):1212–9.
17. McGirt MJ, Attenello FJ, Atiba A, et al. Symptom recurrence after suboccipital decompression for pediatric Chiari I malformation: analysis of 256 consecutive cases. Childs Nerv Syst 2008;24:1333–9.
18. Meadows J, Kraut M, Guarnieri M, et al. Asymptomatic Chiari Type I malformations identified on magnetic resonance imaging. J Neurosurg 2000;92(6): 920–6.
19. Mendes GA, Dickman CA, Rodriguez-Martinez NG, et al. Endoscopic endonasal atlantoaxial transarticular screw fixation technique: an anatomical feasibility and biomechanical study. J Neurosurg Spine 2015; 22(5):470–7.
20. Menezes AH. Acquired abnormalities of the craniovertebral junction. In: Winn HR, editor. Youman's neurological surgery. Philadelphia: Saunders; 2003. p. 4569–85.
21. Tubbs RS, Beckman J, Naftel RP, et al. Institutional experience with 500 cases of surgically treated pediatric Chiari malformation type I. J Neurosurg Pediatr 2011;7:248–56.
22. Yu Y, Hu F, Zhang X, et al. Endoscopic transnasal odontoidectomy combined with posterior reduction to treat basilar invagination: technical note. J Neurosurg Spine 2013;19(5):637–43.
23. Menezes AH. Craniovertebral junction database analysis: incidence, classification, presentation, and treatment algorithms. Childs Nerv Syst 2008; 24(10):1101–8.
24. Menezes AH. Decision making. Childs Nerv Syst 2008;24(10):1147–53.
25. Dlouhy BJ, Dahdaleh NS, Menezes AH. Evolution of transoral approaches, endoscopic endonasal approaches, and reduction strategies for treatment of craniovertebral junction pathology: a treatment algorithm update. Neurosurg Focus 2015;38(4):E8.
26. Henn JS, Lee MC, Rhoton AL. Transoral approach to the craniocervical junction and upper cervical spine. In: Surgical anatomy and techniques of the spine. 1st edition. Philadelphia: Elsevier; 2006. p. 3–12.
27. Singh H, Harrop J, Schiffmacher P, et al. Ventral surgical approaches to craniovertebral junction chordomas. Neurosurgery 2010;66(3 Suppl):96–103.
28. Hickman ZL, McDowell MM, Barton SM, et al. Transnasal endoscopic approach to the pediatric craniovertebral junction and rostral cervical spine: case series and literature review. Neurosurg Focus 2013;35(2):E14.

Spinal Deformity Associated with Chiari Malformation

Michael P. Kelly, MD, MSc[a],*, Tenner J. Guillaume, MD[b],
Lawrence G. Lenke, MD[a]

KEYWORDS

- Scoliosis • Chiari malformation • Syrinx • Syringomyelia • Early onset

KEY POINTS

- Scoliosis commonly occurs in the setting of Chiari I malformation (CM) and even more frequently in the setting of CM with syringomyelia.
- Decompression of the CM is often recommended because it may lead to resolution of the spinal deformity and may make any subsequent spinal deformity surgery safer.
- Spinal deformities are more likely to improve after CM decompression in young patients (<10 years) with small coronal Cobb measurements (<30°).
- Spinal deformity surgery may be more challenging in these patients, in part because of difficulties with intraoperative neurologic monitoring challenges.
- Despite the frequency of this disease process, the pathophysiology remains poorly understood.

INTRODUCTION

Scoliosis is associated with the presence of a Chiari I malformation (CM) in up to 20% of patients, and even more frequently associated with CM in the setting of syringomyelia, with rates as high as 60%. Although this clinical entity is not particularly rare in practice, there is a paucity of published research regarding spinal deformities associated with CM. Thus, the pathophysiology of the spinal deformity, and the effects of the CM with or without syringomyelia, remain poorly understood. Some clinicians have proposed that the formation of a syrinx may cause anterior horn cell dysfunction, with scoliosis as a result.[1,2] Because syringomyelia is not necessary for concomitant scoliosis, other clinicians have proposed that cerebellar tonsil compression is the inciting event.[3] However, identifying patients with this constellation of diagnoses is essential, because there may be some neurologic risk to corrective surgery for the spinal deformity performed in the setting of an untreated syrinx or CM. Furthermore, early diagnosis of scoliosis associated with CM may allow for nonoperative management of the spinal deformity, thus avoiding a spinal fusion.[4–6] This article reviews the current literature regarding scoliosis associated with CM, with and without syringomyelia.

CLINICAL PRESENTATION

The presentation of scoliosis associated with CM varies significantly and, as such, it may remain undiagnosed, so spine surgeons should have some clinical suspicion when evaluating idiopathic

Disclosure: See last page of the article.
[a] Department of Orthopedic Surgery, Washington University School of Medicine, 660 South Euclid Avenue, Box 8233, Saint Louis, MO 63110, USA; [b] Department of Orthopedic Surgery, Gillette Children's Hospital, 200 University Ave E, St Paul, MN 55101, USA
* Corresponding author.
E-mail address: kellymi@wudosis.wustl.edu

scoliosis that shows any atypical features. Charry and colleagues[7] reported a series of patient with syringomyelia in whom a small number had abnormal examinations (10 out of 25; 40%) and most were normal. Up to 10% of patients with suspected idiopathic scoliosis had some abnormality on preoperative MRI, most of which were syringomyelia (67%) followed by Chiari malformations (31%).[8] However, a prospective, observational cohort of patients aged 10 to 19 years did not support these findings, and the clinical concern from disease presentation and physical examination findings are likely the most important factors.[9,10] The diagnosis of scoliosis made in childhood is categorized by age, with children diagnosed as having infantile (birth to 3 years old), juvenile (4–10 years), and adolescent (>10 years old) scoliosis. The age of the child is important to consider, because young cases (infantile and juvenile, early onset scoliosis) of scoliosis are more frequently associated with some neural axis abnormality and an MRI study of the entire spine must be ordered.[11–13] Age and skeletal maturity are important considerations, not only as predictors of the presence of a neural axis abnormality but also because there are implications for prognosis and potential for resolution with management of the CM and syrinx.[4,5,14–16] Menarchal status is assessed in girls, because this may correlate with curve progression and allows for a more informed conversation with patient and parents.[17]

In some cases, neurologic symptoms may precede the diagnosis of the spinal deformity. Perhaps the most common neurologic complaint is headaches, but sensory or motor disturbances may exist.[18] The presence of any of these in an orthopedic clinic should elicit an MRI study of the entire spinal column, with referral to a neurosurgeon should the MRI find abnormalities. A complete neurologic examination must be performed at the initial visit for any child presenting with a spinal deformity. In many cases the examination is normal; however, in some instances a motor deficit, hyperreflexia, or a pathologic reflex may be present. Among the reflexes that must be examined are the abdominal reflexes, because these have been correlated with neural axis abnormalities, including syringomyelia.[19,20] Gait should be examined and clonus should be checked to ensure symmetry and that there are no more than 2 to 3 beats per side, if present at all. Patients presenting as adults may have more profound neurologic abnormalities, which should prompt MRI before any surgical intervention for the spinal deformity.[21]

RADIOGRAPHIC EVALUATION

A standard radiographic evaluation of spinal deformity includes upright, posteroanterior, and lateral full-spine images. The most commonly used classification system for adolescent idiopathic scoliosis (AIS) is the Lenke classification.[22] The usual AIS deformity is an apex right, main thoracic curve, with a loss of thoracic kyphosis at the apex of the deformity (Fig. 1). Atypical findings on posteroanterior (coronal plane) radiographs include an apex left thoracic deformity and sharp, angular deformities (Fig. 2A, B).[23] Perhaps the most important detail related to identification of CM is the measurement of the sagittal Cobb angles. In our practice, a Lenke "+" modifier, indicating hyperkyphosis, undergoes MRI to ensure that there is no underlying neurologic abnormality (see Fig. 2C).[5,23,24] In the case of adolescent scoliosis, any atypia to the curve morphology or appearance warrants an MRI examination (see Fig. 2D). As previously noted, early onset scoliosis is more frequently associated with neural axis abnormalities, such as CM.[11,12] Clinicians must remember that a large deformity presenting as AIS was almost certainly present as a juvenile and, in such cases, MRI may be indicated.

Measurement of the coronal Cobb is important for prognostic factors, before decompression of the Chiari malformation. In general terms, the smaller the deformity at the time of presentation, the more likely the patient is to avoid surgery for the spinal deformity.[4,5,15,16] However, risk of spinal deformity progression is multifactorial, and is also related to the skeletal maturity of the patient, which is related to future growth. The Risser score is a reasonable proxy for remaining growth potential and it should be noted on the posteroanterior radiograph, in addition to the descriptives of the spinal deformity itself.[25] Given the varied presentations of these deformities, relationships between the spinal deformity and the underlying CM and syringomyelia have been difficult to describe. Yeom and colleagues[16] and Qiu and colleagues[23] found no relationships between curve magnitude or character and descriptives of tonsillar descent or syrinx character.[16] In contrast, Godzik and colleagues[26] found that larger syringes (maximum diameter >6 mm) were more commonly associated with the presence of a scoliosis. Those patients with severe tonsillar descent (>12 mm) were less likely to have a scoliosis than those with moderate tonsillar descent (5–12 mm). That these findings were not consistent emphasizes the varied nature of presentation and the poorly understood pathophysiology of this disease process.

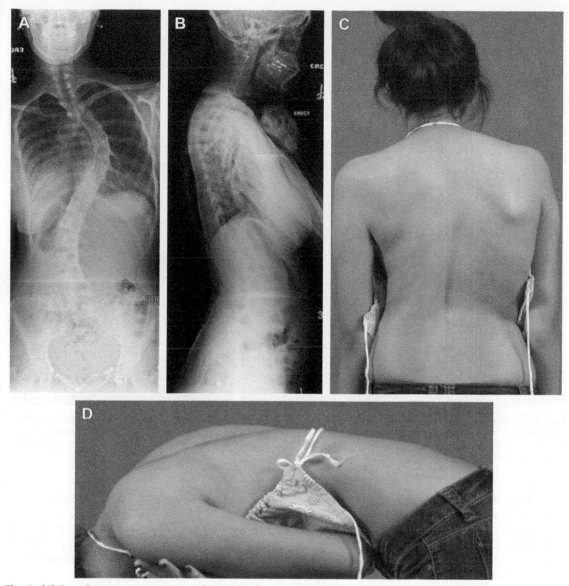

Fig. 1. (*A*) Standing posteroanterior radiograph of a 17-year-old girl with typical radiographic findings of AIS: apex right, no angular deformity. (*B*) Standing lateral radiograph showing thoracic hypokyphosis, typical of AIS. (*C*) Standing clinical image showing a loss of thoracic kyphosis. (*D*) Lateral forward bending clinical image showing a loss of thoracic kyphosis.

MANAGEMENT
Decompression of Chiari

Decompression of the CM may be offered, for both young and old patients, to treat any CM-related symptoms, to potentially minimize the need for future spinal deformity surgery, and to potentially decrease the risk of any future spinal deformity surgery. In young patients (10 years old), there is evidence that decompression of the CM may result in resolution of the spinal deformity, without any further orthopedic intervention.[4,14–16,27,28] Özerdemoglu

and colleagues[29] described their experience, in one of the largest series to date, with 59 patients. Decompression of the hindbrain offered potential benefit to the patients, whereas drainage of a syrinx did not offer any improvements in spinal deformity. Although the pathophysiology remains a debate, there is consistency to the reports of improvement after CM decompression; the deformities tend to be small (<30°) and the patients tend to be young. Brockmeyer and colleagues[15] reported curves as large as 56° improving, although improvement of

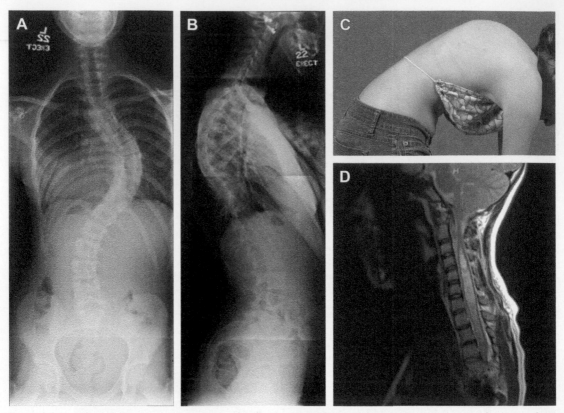

Fig. 2. (*A*) Standing posteroanterior radiograph of a 13-year-old girl with typical coronal plane findings of AIS. (*B*) Standing lateral radiograph showing proximal thoracic kyphosis, atypical for AIS. (*C*) Lateral clinical image of 13-year-old girl with proximal thoracic kyphosis. (*D*) T2-weighted MRI of this young woman, showing Chiari I with syringomyelia.

these large deformities is an exception rather than the rule. Because spontaneous resolution of an idiopathic case of juvenile scoliosis is uncommon, the processes driving these spinal deformities are different in these two types of scoliosis. However, improvements in the deformity are not consistent, and Farley and colleagues[5] reported no improvements in a small series of patients treated with suboccipital decompression and bracing, with 8 of 9 patients requiring spinal fusions.

Decompression is often considered for CM with syringomyelia to potentially reduce the risk of neurologic deficits with surgery. In the absence of a syrinx, the protective benefits of decompression are less compelling, and clinical judgment must be exercised. The presence of a syrinx is more concerning, because lengthening the spinal column through a reduction in the deformity could increase pressure within the fluid column, injuring the neural tissue. The protective benefits of decompression are not known. However, given the potential for catastrophe, it is advisable that the CM be decompressed. Reduction in the syrinx is preferable and reimaging of the spinal column

6 months after the CM decompression is performed to evaluate the status of the syringomyelia. The spine surgeon must know whether a large syrinx exists, both for the preoperative informed decision-making process and for preparation for surgery.

Nonoperative Management

Nonoperative management of scoliosis associated with a CM is similar to management of idiopathic scoliosis, with the exception of the aforementioned neurosurgical intervention. Cases of severe, early onset scoliosis may be managed initially with casting, with transition to bracing or surgical intervention with a growing construct. Nonoperative management of a juvenile or adolescent scoliosis associated with CM is treated with observation for curves smaller than 20°. In skeletally immature patients (eg, Risser stage <4, premenarchal girls) we monitor at 6-month intervals, with a physical examination and standing posteroanterior and lateral full-spine radiographs. Major Cobb angles are compared for evidence of progression. Deformities measuring between 20° and 45° are often treated with a custom-molded thoracolumbosacral orthosis. As with AIS, compliance with brace wear is essential, with a goal of at least 20 hours in the brace per day. Brace wear is continued until the patient has reached skeletal maturity or the curve progresses despite bracing. There is no evidence to support particular nonoperative physical therapy modalities or manipulations in the management of scoliosis associated with CM.

Surgical Management of Spinal Deformity

Indications for surgical intervention in early onset scoliosis associated with CM are similar to those for idiopathic spinal deformities. However, the heterogeneity of spinal deformity makes reliable rules for intervention impossible. In cases in which curves are progressing in spite of casting and bracing, control of the deformity must be obtained to prevent detrimental changes to pulmonary function. A small number of guided-growth techniques exist, including Shilla constructs and growing-rod constructs. CM-associated deformities form a subset of early onset scoliosis worthy of discussion because of the typical curve, hyperkyphotic as opposed to the hypokyphotic scoliosis commonly seen with idiopathic deformities. A growing construct must therefore have control of the deformity in 2 planes, controlling both the progressive kyphosis and scoliosis. In the case of hypokyphosis, control of the scoliosis gives the surgeon adequate control of the sagittal plane deformity, through distraction, and a Shilla procedure may be a reasonable option. In the case of hyperkyphosis, stresses at the proximal end of the construct may be more inclined to loosen, although given the paucity of literature on early onset scoliosis with CM in general there is no peer-reviewed proof of this. For this reason, it may be advisable to performing growing-rod procedures, to obtain control of the proximal segment via fusion with 6 pedicle screws, not 4, again emphasizing a solid grasp of the progressively kyphotic, and growing, proximal segment.

Indications for definitive fusion in older patients are in line with idiopathic recommendations as well. Deformities measuring greater than 50° on upright radiographs are generally considered for surgery. Early reports of spinal fusion in cases of scoliosis associated with CM reported higher rates of perioperative complications.[1] More recent reports have minimized the risk associated with surgery in this patient population, likely because of advances in techniques, instrumentation, imaging, and intraoperative neurologic monitoring. Several series have reported no new neurologic deficits in these surgeries; however, the number of patients examined in these studies is small and the studies may be underpowered to make definitive conclusions regarding safety.[30,31] Each series was complicated by some deformities progressing above or below the fusion levels, stressing the need for careful preoperative evaluation of appropriate construct length. Ferguson and colleagues[30] noted 2 patients developing proximal junctional kyphosis after posterior spinal fusion when the fusion construct was stopped caudal to a prior laminectomy level. We recommend strongly against this and recommend including previously decompressed levels in the fusion construct.

Xie proposed that larger, more severe spinal deformities may not need posterior fossa decompression before spine surgery if a vertebral column resection (VCR) is performed.[32] The VCR shortens the vertebral column and, thus, relaxes the spinal cord. This process decreases tension and pressure within the cord and any syringomyelia that may exist, likely minimizing the risk of iatrogenic injury to the still-compressed hindbrain. However, the VCR is one of the most dangerous and technically challenging procedures performed by pediatric spinal deformity surgeons, with intraoperative neurologic event rates (spinal cord monitoring change or new neurologic deficit) approaching 30% in one series.[33] Thus, clinicians must weigh the potential risks and benefits of VCR versus a staged decompression and posterior spinal fusion in scoliosis associated with CM.

The consideration of VCR for management of scoliosis associated with CM raises an important technical consideration, which is the use intraoperative neurophysiologic monitoring (IOM). IOM is mandatory in any spinal deformity surgery. Commonly used modalities include somatosensory evoked potentials and transcranial motor evoked potentials (TcMEP). These methods monitor the posterior column sensory tracts and anterior column motor tracts, respectively. A less common modality is neurogenic motor evoked potentials, which monitor sensory pathways in an antidromic fashion and may serve as an alternative to TcMEP. Because IOM is an imperfect modality, patients should be instructed on the Stagnara intraoperative wake-up test and be prepared to perform a rehearsed examination should difficulties with IOM data arise.[34] Our experience emphasizes this, because we have found more frequent IOM difficulties with chiari-associated spinal deformities than with AIS (27% vs 3%; $P = .007$). Xie and colleagues did not sustain any neurologic deficits in their VCR series, although these surgeries were performed without IOM and this is unadvisable.

SUMMARY

Despite the frequency of Chiari-associated spinal deformities, this disease process remains poorly understood. Syringomyelia is often present; however, this is not a necessary situation and scoliosis has been described in the absence of a syrinx. Decompression of the hindbrain may be considered but the protective benefits remain unclear. In young patients (<10 years old) and/or those with small coronal Cobb measurements (<40°), decompression of the hindbrain may lead to resolution of the spinal deformity. Spinal fusion is reserved for those curves that progress to deformities greater than 50°. These procedures may be associated with a higher risk of postoperative deficit and intraoperative neurologic monitoring may be difficult. Patients, families, and surgeons should be prepared for this possibility. Further research is needed to understand the underlying pathophysiology to improve prognostication and treatment of this patient population.

DISCLOSURE

Dr M.P. Kelly receives research funding from AOSpine, Orthopedic Research and Education Foundation, Barnes Jewish Foundation, and the Cervical Spine Research Society. Dr L.G. Lenke shares numerous patents with Medtronic (unpaid). He receives substantial royalties from Medtronic and modest royalties from Quality Medical Publishing. Dr L.G. Lenke also receives or has received reimbursement related to meetings/courses from AMCICO, AOSpine, COA, BroadWater, DePuy, Dubai Spine Society, Medtronic, SOSORT, The Spinal Research Foundation, SRS and SSF. This project was supported by the Clinical and Translational Science Award (CTSA) program of the National Center for Advancing Translational Sciences of the National Institutes of Health (NIH) under Award Number UL1 TR000448.

REFERENCES

1. Huebert HT, MacKinnon WB. Syringomyelia and scoliosis. J Bone Joint Surg Br 1969;51:338–43.
2. Isu T, Iwasaki Y, Akino M, et al. Hydrosyringomyelia associated with a Chiari I malformation in children and adolescents. Neurosurgery 1990;26:591–6 [discussion: 596–7].
3. Brockmeyer DL. Editorial. Chiari malformation Type I and scoliosis: the complexity of curves. J Neurosurg Pediatr 2011;7:22–3 [discussion: 23–4].
4. Eule JM, Erickson MA, O'Brien MF, et al. Chiari I malformation associated with syringomyelia and scoliosis: a twenty-year review of surgical and nonsurgical treatment in a pediatric population. Spine (Phila Pa 1976) 2002;27:1451–5.
5. Farley FA, Puryear A, Hall JM, et al. Curve progression in scoliosis associated with Chiari I malformation following suboccipital decompression. J Spinal Disord Tech 2002;15:410–4.
6. Krieger MD, Falkinstein Y, Bowen IE, et al. Scoliosis and Chiari malformation Type I in children. J Neurosurg Pediatr 2011;7:25–9.
7. Charry O, Koop S, Winter R, et al. Syringomyelia and scoliosis: a review of twenty-five pediatric patients. J Pediatr Orthop 1994;14:309–17.
8. Diab M, Landman Z, Lubicky J, et al. Use and outcome of MRI in the surgical treatment of adolescent idiopathic scoliosis. Spine (Phila Pa 1976) 2011;36:667–71.
9. Do T, Fras C, Burke S, et al. Clinical value of routine preoperative magnetic resonance imaging in adolescent idiopathic scoliosis. A prospective study of three hundred and twenty-seven patients. J Bone Joint Surg Am 2001;83-A:577–9.
10. Davids JR, Chamberlin E, Blackhurst DW. Indications for magnetic resonance imaging in presumed adolescent idiopathic scoliosis. J Bone Joint Surg Am 2004;86-A:2187–95.
11. Gupta P, Lenke LG, Bridwell KH. Incidence of neural axis abnormalities in infantile and juvenile patients with spinal deformity. Is a magnetic resonance image screening necessary? Spine (Phila Pa 1976) 1998;23:206–10.
12. Dobbs MB, Lenke LG, Szymanski DA, et al. Prevalence of neural axis abnormalities in patients with infantile idiopathic scoliosis. J Bone Joint Surg Am 2002;84-A:2230–4.
13. Koc T, Lam KS, Webb JK. Are intraspinal anomalies in early onset idiopathic scoliosis as common as once thought? A two centre United Kingdom study. Eur Spine J 2013;22:1250–4.
14. Attenello FJ, McGirt MJ, Atiba A, et al. Suboccipital decompression for Chiari malformation-associated scoliosis: risk factors and time course of deformity progression. J Neurosurg Pediatr 2008;1:456–60.
15. Brockmeyer D, Gollogly S, Smith JT. Scoliosis associated with Chiari 1 malformations: the effect of suboccipital decompression on scoliosis curve progression: a preliminary study. Spine (Phila Pa 1976) 2003;28:2505–9.
16. Yeom JS, Lee C-K, Park K-W, et al. Scoliosis associated with syringomyelia: analysis of MRI and curve progression. Eur Spine J 2007;16:1629–35.
17. Little DG, Song KM, Katz D, et al. Relationship of peak height velocity to other maturity indicators in idiopathic scoliosis in girls. J Bone Joint Surg Am 2000;82:685–93.
18. Hida K, Iwasaki Y, Koyanagi I, et al. Pediatric syringomyelia with Chiari malformation: its clinical

characteristics and surgical outcomes. Surg Neurol 1999;51:383–90 [discussion: 390–1].

19. Nakahara D, Yonezawa I, Kobanawa K, et al. Magnetic resonance imaging evaluation of patients with idiopathic scoliosis: a prospective study of four hundred seventy-two outpatients. Spine (Phila Pa 1976) 2011;36:E482–5.

20. Zadeh HG, Sakka SA, Powell MP, et al. Absent superficial abdominal reflexes in children with scoliosis. An early indicator of syringomyelia. J Bone Joint Surg Br 1995;77:762–7.

21. Ono A, Suetsuna F, Ueyama K, et al. Surgical outcomes in adult patients with syringomyelia associated with Chiari malformation type I: the relationship between scoliosis and neurological findings. J Neurosurg Spine 2007;6:216–21.

22. Lenke LG, Betz RR, Harms J, et al. Adolescent idiopathic scoliosis: a new classification to determine extent of spinal arthrodesis. J Bone Joint Surg Am 2001;83-A:1169–81.

23. Qiu Y, Zhu Z, Wang B, et al. Radiological presentations in relation to curve severity in scoliosis associated with syringomyelia. J Pediatr Orthop 2008;28: 128–33.

24. Whitaker C, Schoenecker PL, Lenke LG. Hyperkyphosis as an indicator of syringomyelia in idiopathic scoliosis: a case report. Spine (Phila Pa 1976) 2003; 28:E16–20.

25. Noordeen MH, Haddad FS, Edgar MA, et al. Spinal growth and a histologic evaluation of the Risser grade in idiopathic scoliosis. Spine (Phila Pa 1976) 1999;24:535–8.

26. Godzik J, Kelly MP, Radmanesh A, et al. Relationship of syrinx size and tonsillar descent to spinal deformity in Chiari malformation Type I with associated syringomyelia. J Neurosurg Pediatr 2014;13:368–74.

27. Sengupta DK, Dorgan J, Findlay GF. Can hindbrain decompression for syringomyelia lead to regression of scoliosis? Eur Spine J 2000;9:198–201.

28. Hwang SW, Samdani AF, Jea A, et al. Outcomes of Chiari I-associated scoliosis after intervention: a meta-analysis of the pediatric literature. Childs Nerv Syst 2012;28:1213–9.

29. Özerdemoglu RA, Transfeldt EE, Denis F. Value of treating primary causes of syrinx in scoliosis associated with syringomyelia. Spine 2003;28:806–14.

30. Ferguson RL, Devine J, Stasikelis P, et al. Outcomes in surgical treatment of " idiopathic-like" scoliosis associated with syringomyelia. J Spinal Disord Tech 2002;15:301–6.

31. Bradley LJ, Ratahi ED, Crawford HA, et al. The outcomes of scoliosis surgery in patients with syringomyelia. Spine 2007;32:2327–33.

32. Xie J, Wang Y, Zhao Z, et al. One-stage and posterior approach for correction of moderate to severe scoliosis in adolescents associated with Chiari I malformation: is a prior suboccipital decompression always necessary? Eur Spine J 2011;20:1106–13.

33. Lenke LG, Newton PO, Sucato DJ, et al. Complications after 147 consecutive vertebral column resections for severe pediatric spinal deformity: a multicenter analysis. Spine (Phila Pa 1976) 2013; 38:119–32.

34. Wilson-Holden TJ, Padberg AM, Lenke LG, et al. Efficacy of intraoperative monitoring for pediatric patients with spinal cord pathology undergoing spinal deformity surgery. Spine (Phila Pa 1976) 1999;24: 1685–92.

Index

Note: Page numbers of article titles are in **boldface.**

United States Postal Service

Statement of Ownership, Management, and Circulation
(All Periodicals Publications Except Requester Publications)

1. Publication Title — Neurosurgery Clinics of North America
2. Publication Number — 0 1 0 - 5 4 8
3. Filing Date — 9/18/15

4. Issue Frequency — Jan, Apr, Jul, Oct
5. Number of Issues Published Annually — 4
6. Annual Subscription Price — $380.00

7. Complete Mailing Address of Known Office of Publication (Not printer) (Street, city, county, state, and ZIP+4®)

Elsevier Inc.
360 Park Avenue South
New York, NY 10010-1710

Contact Person — Stephen R. Bushing

Telephone (Include area code) — 215-239-3688

8. Complete Mailing Address of Headquarters or General Business Office of Publisher (Not printer)

Elsevier Inc., 360 Park Avenue South, New York, NY 10010-1710

9. Full Names and Complete Mailing Addresses of Publisher, Editor, and Managing Editor (Do not leave blank)

Publisher (Name and complete mailing address)

Linda Belfus, Elsevier Inc., 1600 John F. Kennedy Blvd., Suite 1800, Philadelphia, PA 19103

Editor (Name and complete mailing address)

Jennifer Flynn-Briggs, Elsevier Inc., 1600 John F. Kennedy Blvd., Suite 1800, Philadelphia, PA 19103-2899

Managing Editor (Name and complete mailing address)

Adrianne Brigido, Elsevier Inc., 1600 John F. Kennedy Blvd., Suite 1800, Philadelphia, PA 19103-2899

10. Owner (Do not leave blank. If the publication is owned by a corporation, give the name and address of the corporation immediately followed by the names and addresses of all stockholders owning or holding 1 percent or more of the total amount of stock. If not owned by a corporation, give the names and addresses of the individual owners. If owned by a partnership or other unincorporated firm, give its name and address as well as those of each individual owner. If the publication is published by a nonprofit organization, give its name and address.)

Full Name	Complete Mailing Address
Wholly owned subsidiary of	1600 John F. Kennedy Blvd., Ste. 1800
Reed/Elsevier, US holdings	Philadelphia, PA 19103-2899

11. Known Bondholders, Mortgagees, and Other Security Holders Owning or Holding 1 Percent or More of Total Amount of Bonds, Mortgages, or Other Securities. If none, check box ☐ None

Full Name	Complete Mailing Address
N/A	

12. Tax Status (For completion by nonprofit organizations authorized to mail at nonprofit rates) (Check one)
The purpose, function, and nonprofit status of this organization and the exempt status for federal income tax purposes:
☐ Has Not Changed During Preceding 12 Months
☐ Has Changed During Preceding 12 Months (Publisher must submit explanation of change with this statement)

13. Publication Title — Neurosurgery Clinics of North America

14. Issue Date for Circulation Data Below — July 2015

PS Form 3526, July 2014 (Page 1 of 3 (Instructions Page 3)) PSN 7530-01-000-9931 PRIVACY NOTICE: See our Privacy policy in www.usps.com

15. Extent and Nature of Circulation			Average No. Copies Each Issue During Preceding 12 Months	No. Copies of Single Issue Published Nearest to Filing Date
a. Total Number of Copies (Net press run)			511	489
b. Legitimate Paid and Or Requested Distribution (By Mail and Outside the Mail)	(1)	Mailed Outside-County Paid/Requested Mail Subscriptions stated on PS Form 3541. (Include paid distribution above nominal rate, advertiser's proof copies and exchange copies)	150	126
	(2)	Mailed In-County Paid/Requested Mail Subscriptions stated on PS Form 3541. (Include paid distribution above nominal rate, advertiser's proof copies and exchange copies)		
	(3)	Paid Distribution Outside the Mails Including Sales Through Dealers And Carriers, Street Vendors, Counter Sales, and Other Paid Distribution Outside USPS®	81	90
	(4)	Paid Distribution by Other Classes of Mail Through the USPS (e.g. First-Class Mail®)		
c. Total Paid and or Requested Circulation (Sum of 15b (1), (2), (3), and (4))			231	216
d. Free or Nominal Rate Distribution (By Mail and Outside the Mail)	(1)	Free or Nominal Rate Outside-County Copies included on PS Form 3541	76	59
	(2)	Free or Nominal Rate In-County Copies included on PS Form 3541		
	(3)	Free or Nominal Rate Copies mailed at Other classes Through the USPS (e.g. First-Class Mail®)		
	(4)	Free or Nominal Rate Distribution Outside the Mail (Carriers or Other means)		
e. Total Nonrequested Distribution (Sum of 15d (1), (2), (3) and (4)			76	59
f. Total Distribution (Sum of 15c and 15e)			307	275
g. Copies not Distributed (See instructions to publishers #4 (page #3))			204	214
h. Total (Sum of 15f and g)			511	489
i. Percent Paid and/or Requested Circulation (15c divided by 15f times 100)			75.24%	78.55%

* If you are claiming electronic copies go to line 16 on page 3. If you are not claiming Electronic copies, skip to line 17 on page 3.

16. Electronic Copy Circulation	Average No. Copies Each Issue During Preceding 12 Months	No. Copies of Single Issue Published Nearest to Filing Date
a. Paid Electronic Copies		
b. Total paid Print Copies (Line 15c) + Paid Electronic copies (Line 16a)		
c. Total Print Distribution (Line 15f) + Paid Electronic Copies (Line 16a)		
d. Percent Paid (Both Print & Electronic copies) (16b divided by 16c X 100)		

☐ I certify that 50% of all my distributed copies (electronic and print) are paid above a nominal price

17. Publication of Statement of Ownership
If the publication is a general publication, publication of this statement is required. Will be printed in the **October 2015** issue of this publication.

18. Signature and Title of Editor, Publisher, Business Manager, or Owner — Date — September 18, 2015

Stephen R. Bushing

Stephen R. Bushing – Inventory Distribution Coordinator

I certify that all information furnished on this form is true and complete. I understand that anyone who furnishes false or misleading information on this form or who omits material or information requested on the form may be subject to criminal sanctions (including fines and imprisonment) and/or civil sanctions (including civil penalties).

PS Form 3526, July 2014 (Page 3 of 3)

Printed and bound by CPI Group (UK) Ltd, Croydon, CR0 4YY

03/10/2024

01040366-0004